Eating for Two

EATING FOR TWO

Recipes for *Pregnant and Breastfeeding Women*

Robin Lim

CELESTIAL ARTS
Berkeley | Toronto

Celestial Arts
P.O. Box 7123
Berkeley, California 94707
www.tenspeed.com

Distributed in Australia by Simon and Schuster Australia, in Canada by Ten Speed Press Canada, in New Zealand by Southern Publishers Group, in South Africa by Real Books, and in the United Kingdom and Europe by Airlift Book Company.

Cover design by Susanne Weihl

Interior design by Lynn Bell, Monroe Street Studios, Santa Rosa, California

Library of Congress Cataloging-in-Publication Data
Lim, Robin, 1956–
  Eating for two : recipes for pregnant and breastfeeding women / Robin Lim.
    p. cm.
Includes index.
  ISBN 1-58761-182-1
  1. Pregnancy—Nutritional aspects. 2. Lactation—Nutritional aspects. 3. Cookery. I. Title.
RG559.L56 2003
618.2'4—dc22

                                    2003022475

First printing, 2003

Printed in the United States

1 2 3 4 5 6 7 8 9 10 — 06 05 04 03

To the mothers of our world

ACKNOWLEDGMENTS

All projects require vision, courage, enthusiasm, and action. The people I wish to honor have shared with me these four precious and necessary ingredients. If there were a recipe for becoming a healer, the first ingredient would be support—from family, friends, and the community. In the years of gathering knowledge and recipes for this book my family has been sheltered by the aloha of Maui, Hawaii; Fairfield, Iowa; Baguio City, Philippine Islands; and Nyuh Kuning village in Bali, Indonesia. Mahalo. Thank you. Maraming salamat. Terima kasih banyak.

This book represents a passion for maternal health and infant survival nurtured by the following midwives: June Whitson and Sunny Supplee, both missed on this Earth and relied upon in spirit. The living midwives who have nourished me include: Jan Francisco, Tina Garzero, Jeannine Parvati Baker (high priestess in the religion of Gratitude), Jan Tritten, Debby Lowry, Mary Jackson, Joanne Dugas, Ina May Gaskin, Anne Frye, Nan Koehler, Yeshi Neumann, Jenna Houston, Pearl Breitbach, Kathy Deol, Diana Runyan, Kate Bowland, Roxanne Potter, Melody Weig, Beverly Francis, Marina Alzugaray, Sandra Morningstar, Dorisse Neale, Kadi Mourningstar, Stephanie Struthmann, Kalanete, Nancy Wainer, Valerie El Halta, Faith Gibson, Mary Offerman, Rahima Baldwin, Elizabeth Davis, Linda Harrison, Raven Lang, Lori Arak, and Pamela Hunt.

On my knees I thank the following women who have helped me receive babies in Bali: Ibu June, Mary Kroeger (my heart's right hand), Dr. Eden Gabrielle Fromberg, Dr. Injil Abu Bakar, Gina Catena, Ibu Puthri, Elaine Mellon, Lauren Drescher, Ni Ketut Rusni, Ni Wayan Liwati, Brenda Ritchmond, and my daughter Zhou Lee.

The doulas, who mother the mothers, and who nurtured this book: Marci Freeman, Debra Pascali-Bonaro, Joanne Poole, Dr. Lynne Walker, Olivia Winter, Toni Sugg, Christina Wadsworth, and that wise woman in the North, Marie Zenack.

Recipes for food and songs for good living were contributed by the above named as well as Hannelore Josam, Christine Goodale, Debby Nofthaft, Marcello Pietrobon, Rebecca Bashara and Scott MacDonald, Megan Robinson, Sophia Anastasia, Judy Smith and David Oye, Marjan DeJong,

Alesia Lloyd, Gina and Steve Sitz, Wayan Sudarmi, Katie and Tim Britton, Rick Stanley, Pat Egan, Steve Jakamini, Phyllis Gurchinoff, Sandi Coe Neustadt, Kathy Werner, Bruce Grady, Remy Lim, Monet Lim, Angie Lim Baker, Amalia Bright, Dawn Wiederman, Carole Montanari, Marina and Joseph Yacoe, Rusni and Sam Shapiro, Pak Frank Wilson, Caree Connet, Alloysha, Deja Bernhardt, Frank Wilson, Rosie Estrin, Lonica and Michael Halley, Cindy Miller, Martha Sperry, Rebecca Hougher, Christy Lord Hartridge, Debra Brittingham, Diane Frank, Nancy Cook, Kelly Miller, Aleshanee Akin, Andy Carmone and Sarthak Das, John Briley M.D., Dr. Jon Estrin, Linda and Babu Walling, Suzanne Arms, Margo Berdeshevsky, Priya and Pradheep Chhalliyil, Anjalie Trice, Aron Keuhneumann, Ivana Kurtz, Julan and Bonnie White, Alex Green for great tofu, Sivan Wind, Jaladeen for garden seeds, The Polack family, the late Chrissy Walker, *Midwifery Today,* Bali Buddha, Brenda Ritchmond, Maj Nathanson, and Everybody at Everybody's Health Food Store.

At Celestial Arts I am blessed to hold hands with the late and ever appreciated David Hinds, Annie Nelson (midwife to this book), Kirsty Melville, and Brook Barnum, head roustabout.

At the feet of my spiritual mother, Mata Amritanandamayi—who is living hope that the womanly way of the "Mother" will heal our world—I place this book.

To my own mother, Cresencia Lim Jehle; and my dear late father, Robert A. Jehle; my brothers, Bob, Carl, and Gregory; and my sister, Christine, my angel, words cannot express my gratitude. My lola, Vicenta Lim; gets a special mention for all the ways she nourished the little midwife in me as I was growing up.

In the religion of Gratitude, my husband, Wil, is the choirmaster, high priest, and chief taste tester. My children, Déjà, Noël, Zhòu, Lakota, Zion, Thoreau, and Hanoman, and granddaughter, Zhouie, are the Buddhas my heart sings to. Has any of you seen my measuring spoons?

Contents

FOREWORD

Imagine sitting in your best friend's kitchen while she prepares a meal for you. Children play in the background, bringing a bunch of herbs or edible flowers from the garden, or a new picture to hang on the refrigerator. Now imagine that your best friend is a midwife, and that you are pregnant. The food she lovingly prepares awakens your senses and nurtures you and your baby. Your body is optimally nourished to cope with the changes and challenges of pregnancy and breastfeeding as you and your baby grow strong and healthy.

Robin Lim's wonderful book *Eating for Two: Recipes for Pregnant and Breastfeeding Women* brings the midwife into your kitchen. Robin's wisdom and caring shines through these pages as she weaves sound nutritional recommendations together with delicious recipes that support health and life. Even before reading the recipes, flip to the back of the book and read the afterword: "Who Is Robin Lim? And Why Is She Writing a Cookbook?" Better you find out now so that you can even more thoroughly enjoy the multicultural cast of family, friends, birthing families, and midwife sisters contributing to the range of recipes found within.

Pregnancy and breastfeeding are nutritionally demanding times in a woman's life, and are particularly vulnerable to the effects of nutritional imbalance. As the growing baby and placenta adapt in an attempt to compensate for any prenatal nutritional imbalances, irreversible developmental changes known as "metabolic programming" occur. Ongoing research has linked prenatal nutritional imbalances to problems ranging from neural tube defects, low birth weight, cognitive delays, and obesity to the development of chronic disease—including high blood pressure, cardiovascular disease, type II diabetes, and osteoporosis. Environmental pesticides and petrochemicals act as "xenobiotics," mimicking hormones within our bodies and leading to hormonal imbalance, reproductive abnormalities, infertility, and cancer. Robin recommends choosing organically grown food, which contains considerably lower levels of xenobiotics. Genetically engineered foods have only recently been introduced into our food supply. Read Robin's compelling information on why to avoid them. These issues are of broad significance, affecting the health of women and children worldwide.

Additionally, the American Academy of Pediatrics advocates breastfeeding as the optimal, uniquely superior form of nutrition for all infants. Breast-feeding enhances cognitive development and intelligence, and decreases the incidence and severity of allergies as well as numerous acute and chronic ill-nesses. Women who breastfeed will be rewarded with a more rapid return to prepregnancy weight, and lower risks of osteoporosis, breast cancer, and ovarian cancer.

Sound nutrition is essential to life, and even more so to the creation and nurturing of new life. As self-evident as this may seem, in my own practice as an obstetrician/gynecologist, it is apparent that many women are con-fused about healthy eating. Conflicting and often inaccurate messages from the media and culture further confuse the issue. Studies have shown that the development of a negative body image due to societal messages that favor thinness begins in girls as young as six years old, if not earlier, and correlates with the number of hours of television watched per week. "Diets" are generally conducted for the purpose of losing weight. Women are frequently accustomed to restricting calories, dangerously skimping on nutrition as a result, and some women have eating disorders that lead to even more severe nutritional imbalances. Those who eat "well" may in fact be consuming excess sugar, calories, and fat, but lacking essential protein, vitamins, and minerals. The truth is that healthy eating habits and food choices constitute the best "diet" for maintaining normal body weight, and a healthy and nutritious diet promotes a healthy body, regardless of size or shape. Good nutrition is a lifelong, intergenerational process that directly affects health and well being. A mother who eats and prepares nutritious food will positively influence the health of her entire family. Preparing for conception and becoming pregnant is an excellent motivation for women to assess their food and lifestyle choices and make healthy changes. Robin offers practical information and advice, and nutritious, delicious, family-tested recipes that are easy and fun to prepare. And eat!

Whether in Bali or in Iowa, Robin's kitchen is always a warm, fragrant, welcoming center of activity. People really do drop by, all the time. And there's always a handful of almonds, a cup of tea, a bowl of yellow rice, and a birthday dinner fit for a queen. I was fortunate enough to be in Robin's kitchen in Bali when Iskandar's Asparagus Spread (page 209) was conceived. Two days after Robin's Thanksgiving birthday feast, the day after receiving Ade's baby, I sat at Robin's kitchen table, glazed over in the tropical heat. Ade's brother, Iskandar, an organic farmer, had dropped off a big basket of asparagus that morning. Robin looked up from a blender full of creamy green puree she had been working on. "Eden," she said, "you are not going to believe this asparagus stuff!" It wasn't long before we were spooning the spread onto the only bagels in Bali (baked locally at Bali Buddha, with Robin's recipe, of course) and licking it off our fingers. It was so good. Robin cooks and experiments with food all the time, and she creates recipes on the spot that she is generous with. Even from Iowa, on the phone to me in New York, Robin will say, "Oh, Sweetie, I wish you were here, I'm making sprouted chickpea falafel, and it smells so good in here—the parents of that beautiful baby I just received brought me a quart of wild blackberries and I'm baking a cobbler." With Robin Lim's *Eating for Two: Recipes for Pregnant and Breastfeeding Women,* we can all visit with and be nourished by the "midwife next door," and create health through good nutrition for ourselves and our families. Enjoy!

Om Shanti,
EDEN GABRIELLE FROMBERG, DO, FACOOG
Clinical Assistant Professor of Obstetrics and Gynecology
Long Island College Hospital, Brooklyn, New York

Making Babies in Increasing Light

Because I was blessed with a daughter while I was still a teenager, my life has been focused on pregnancy, birth, postpartum, breastfeeding, and creating the most amazing family possible. I learned that the care and feeding of children begins before conception. Looking back, I was not nearly as ready to become a mother as I imagined myself to be. However, I was happy and very healthy. I ate excellent, nutritious foods; my environment was clean and wonderful; I spent time outdoors bicycling, swimming, and walking; and I balanced this activity with prenatal yoga, meditation, and rest. The results . . .well, my daughter Déjà is deliciously healthy, strong, intelligent, creative, and beautiful. I went on to mother five children from my body, plus two more I got for "free." Déjà is grown, and herself a mother (my granddaughter is also amazing and healthy). Noël is a tall, healthy young man, nearly twenty-two years old. Zhòu, Lakota, Zion, and Thor are all in their teens (yes, imagine our busy household!); they are growing and glowing. Hanoman, the family fiddler, is nine years old. He was conceived and born in a tiny Balinese village. He's such an unusual child that I wonder if there truly was magic in the red rice and the gamelon music that nourished me during my last pregnancy.

Being a mother and a midwife, I could not help but notice just how important nutritious food prepared with love really is for the growing baby. Healthy mothers have healthy babies: healthy in mind, body, and spirit, too. Likewise the future health of the woman can be greatly enhanced by nutritious, whole foods during and after pregnancy.

Eating wisely during pregnancy lays a strong foundation for our children's bodies. Also remember that it is upon your knee that your babies will learn their future food habits. By modeling a lifestyle of sound nutrition while your children are young, you ensure the health and well-being of your family's future generations.

I've been a mother for twenty-seven years now, and over the course of those years, I've collected and perfected the recipes you'll find in these pages. Though our family normally lives in Asia (Bali, Indonesia, and

Baguio, Philippines), we've had a lovely time in Iowa. Iowa has given me the cold months, during which I gathered my scraps of paper and scribbled recipes. I contacted friends and family and called in all the promised favorite food prescriptions.

In Iowa, around the time of the Winter Solstice, people turn their awareness inward, the work of harvest is behind us, and there is time for gathering around the hearth, making pies, singing, and making babies. By Christmas week I had two calls from couples saying, "We're planning to have a baby. What can we do to help make this a healthy and happy baby?" Christmastime being the season to celebrate birth, I was happy to answer the questions of these families. Indeed, it is always a joy to meet people who wish to consciously conceive. In the wise words of Jeannine Parvati Baker, "Conscious conception is merely a simple yet evocative invitation to participate in a miracle."[1] Even in the busy crunch of what my family calls the "holy daze," I manage to find time to do consultations with couples planning miracles.

By Imbolc (February 2, an ancient Druid holy day) which we remember now as Groundhog Day, when the light ever so slowly increases, the days grow longer, and the world rejoices in the promise of new life, the happy couples had achieved the pregnancies they deeply desired.

By spring . . . Look around. Those blooming apple trees are definitely trying to get pregnant, as are the pear trees. When I sink my fingers into the soil of my garden patch, I can feel "Her" wishing for seeds, for life to spring forth. With the creation of each new life, an opportunity to achieve balance and perfect health from the foundation up presents itself. How to give a new human a beautiful healthy start . . .that is the purpose of this book.

Let's begin with the most basic nutritional advice. We are made of water.[2] One of the most beautiful babies I've ever received was Narayanam, son of Priya. Priya's husband Pradheep was a biochemist with a passion for discovering what increases health; he advised Priya to begin each day with 32 ounces of pure water.[3] To my eyes, all pregnant women glow; however, Priya was virtually a goddess. If you are pregnant or planning to become with child, please drink; in fact, gulp plenty of pure water. Liquids such as sodas and caffeinated drinks do not count.

There is a beautiful Hindu story about the God Brahma, who was asked to give humankind solace from suffering. His gift was simple and beautiful: citrus fruit.

Brahma's son, Narada, was concerned and he questioned his father's wisdom, saying "How can there now be a balance between life and death, production and destruction, when you have given humans the cure for all disease? There will be no illness, no aging, and no death. How can the laws of karma operate without the balance of increasing life, sustaining life, and destroying life?"

"Ah ha!" beamed Brahma. "I am not such a fool. In this miracle citrus fruit I put something that will neutralize its healing properties: the seed. Also, dear son, the seeds of the citrus fruit are small and slippery. Only very wise people will carefully partake of the fruit and avoid the seed.

I retell this story to impress upon expectant parents, and all people, the importance of the gift of citrus fruits. Eat them daily, but don't eat the seeds. Research has proven the power of vitamin C. Did you know that the vitamin C in your body is used up by stress and polluted environments? In our time, it is wise and important to supply your body with plenty of vitamin C, and consider the healing power of getting one's vitamin C right from the source—citrus fruit. My dear friend Sam Shapiro wrote a story entitled, "There's a Cloud in My Tangerine." In this lovely tale, he describes a small girl, who notices when she peels her fruit that a beautiful cloud of aromatic mist rises from her hands. In that cloud she sees the sunshine, the rain, the soil, the farmer who grew the fruit, the cow whose dung fertilized the tree, even the woman who cared for the cow. When eating citrus, and all fruits and vegetables, taste the Earth, the rain, the fire of the sun. Even the wind and the ether is captured in your living food. Just as all the elements participate in the making of a piece of fruit, so, also, are all the elements involved in the creation of a baby.

Eat well and drink plenty; your baby's body will be his or her house, for an entire lifetime. Choose the best-quality organic foods whenever possible; good nutrition is an investment. When people build their dream house, they choose the finest woods; please build your baby's body with as much care.

What about vitamin and mineral supplements? I believe in them because our soil has changed so drastically in the last hundred years. Destructive farming techniques have robbed our soil, and thus our food, of nutrients essential to life. Fortunately there are high-quality, pure vitamin supplements available for pregnant women. Consult with your health care provider about vitamin and mineral supplement choices. I suggest that women seeking to achieve pregnancy begin taking prenatal vitamins and looking toward improving their nutrition, right away.[4]

Also, keep in mind that happiness affects intelligence. We know that the unsaturated fats, or omega oils, inspire brain development. Cortisol, a hormone present in the body in increasing amounts when one is *unhappy*, inhibits the absorption of the unsaturated fats.[5] We can conclude that happy pregnant women are absorbing omega-3 fatty acids more efficiently. The babies of these happy women are getting what they need for optimum brain development. Sadly, unhappy pregnant women have more cortisol present in their bodies, which may inhibit their babies' brain development. When you're pregnant, please . . .don't worry, be happy.

Nutritional sources of the omega oils are flaxseed oil, hemp oil, and sardines. Yes, eat sardines for a smarter baby. According to Dr. Michel Odent, sardines are a deep-water fish, so they are less likely to be polluted, and they provide omega-3 fatty acids, essential to baby's brain development.

Reproduction is nothing short of a miracle. Imagine: conception, pregnancy, birth, lactation . . . these are the steps we take, in partnership with the Divine Maker, to help bring a soul Earth-side. Without a body, a soul has no opportunity to evolve on our beautiful planet. Yes, we live in challenging times, which makes it all the more important to bring souls of increasing light into healthy bodies. We must strive to nurture these Earth-angels in happy families. Maybe, just maybe, one Buddha-full baby at a time, we will create peace on Earth.

[1] Jeannine Parvati Baker and Fredrick Baker, *Conscious Conception Elemental Journey through the Labyrinth of Sexuality* (Berkeley, Ca.: North Atlantic Books or Monroe, Ut.: Freestone Publishing Company 1986, 6th printing 1997), 11.

[2] F. Batmanghelidj, M.D. *Your Body's Many Cries for Water*

[3] www.shakthifoundation.org

[4] My choice of vitamin supplements for expectant mothers is NF Formulas Prenatal Forte.

[5] Michel Odent M.D., "Eat Sardines, Be Happy . . . and Sing!" *Midwifery Today,* Autumn 2001, pg. 19.

INTRODUCTION

Optimal Health Through Nutrition During Pregnancy

Common sense tells us that healthy mothers grow healthy babies. It is also a fact that women who enjoy optimal health have fewer pregnancy discomforts. That is not to say that a woman who experiences nausea during her early pregnancy—or heartburn in later pregnancy—is not healthy. However, a healthy woman can cope more easily with the discomforts. Attention to optimal diet, getting enough rest while remaining active, being happy, and living in a healthy environment, all contribute to a blissful, healthy pregnancy. Attention to your health in pregnancy is the best way to achieve a good and safe birth, as well as a healing, wonderful postpartum. Naturally, your nutrition paves the way for lactation. These are all excellent reasons to eat well, drink plenty, and develop healthy happy habits, today.

Growing a baby is a *job:* twenty-four hours a day, seven days a week. Sadly, in our work a day world, the role of mothering is so diminished that expectant women are not honored as they should be. In my vision of a perfect world, the neighborhood would so celebrate pregnant women that the neighbors would bring special foods, nutritious drinks, and treats daily to the expectant family. In Bali, where I was blessed to be living during my last pregnancy, the women of our village endeavored to feed me. Often, in the early morning, I was presented with a sweet potato pulled right from the hearth fire, the ash lovingly blown off and the warm treasure given right into my hand. Though I was new in the village, these women, who had so little, would bring me steaming bowls of rice gruel with leafy greens to nourish me and my developing baby. Clearly, they loved children so much that they considered each pregnancy a blessing for the entire village. You can see why our family made the village of Nyuh Kuning our home.

In Fairfield, a small town in southeastern Iowa where we often make our home, postpartum women are truly blessed. The community spirit is so strong that, after having a baby, the new mother receives an astonishing gift: Every day, for two to three weeks, her friends deliver nutritious food—enough for the entire family to enjoy lunch and dinner. Is it any wonder that this small town boasts an unusually high rate of breastfeeding? The new mothers are doing exactly what nature intended: they are bonding, resting, and establishing breastfeeding, while their friends do the cooking.

When you are pregnant or postpartum it is the *job* of your family and friends to feed you well. This is the best way to protect your baby's future health and well-being.

My husband, Wil, called my last pregnancy "the mad-scientist experiment." He was determined to make a wonder child—super-happy, super-healthy, super-talented, super-smart, super-creative. He took over the shopping, juiced vegetables and fruits for me, and cooked excellent meals for our entire family. Unfortunately, I could hardly appreciate his efforts, as I had intense nausea, so for my comfort he massaged me. To increase my happiness, Wil sang songs with the children every evening at bedtime. The results . . . well, our son Hanoman turned out to be a redhead! He's healthy, vibrant, climbs like a monkey, and is musical—an all-around amazing boy. The point of the story is that we nourished my body, heart, mind, and soul while I was expecting, and our child got off to a fabulous start. Because I was healthy and felt safe, Hanoman's birth was wrinkle-free. Because he's had a healthy start, this boy is free to grow up strong and well. Believe me, it is a joy to witness.

WHAT ABOUT WEIGHT GAIN?

Women eating and drinking well while getting plenty of rest and activity during pregnancy need not worry about weight gain. Please, do not for any reason diet for weight loss during pregnancy. Dieting is dangerous and can lead to low birth-weight babies. Keep in mind that weight gain in pregnancy is necessary for the health of your baby. At term, approximately one-quarter of your weight gain is the baby. Three-quarters of the weight you gain during pregnancy is additional blood volume, placenta, amniotic and other fluids, fat for protective cushioning, and additional tissue in your uterus and breasts.

During the first three months of pregnancy many women experience bouts of nausea and vomiting. Also, during this first trimester, you do need approximately 100 *additional* calories per day. Yet, you need not worry if you are vomiting, as 100 calories is not that much. (If you are vomiting very often, you must consult your midwife or doctor.) The quality of the food you eat is more important than the quantity. By choosing nutritious, organic, lovingly prepared whole foods, you are making every bite count. By the last trimester, when you need approximately 400 additional calories per day, you will feel less nausea and keep your food down like most women do.

You can expect to gain between 25 and 35 pounds during your pregnancy. Any gradual weight gain is normal: even if you gradually gain more than 35 pounds, don't be afraid. The extra stored calories will come in handy when you are breastfeeding. If you began your pregnancy while underweight, you may very well gain more than the average. Again, don't be alarmed. I repeat, do not diet. Weight gain is individual. Your job is not to count calories. Instead you must eat wholesome foods so that every calorie adds up to good nutrition.

PROTEIN

Every cell in your baby's developing body is built with protein. You also need protein so that your blood volume and new tissues will increase. To build a house you need wood; to build a baby, you must have protein. I ask my pregnant women to supply their bodies with a minimum of two servings of about 15 grams of protein or more, per day. Morning and evening you must eat protein. The following is a list[1] of protein sources, each of which adds up to approximately 15 grams:

Eggs: 2 large
Tofu: ¾ cup
Tempeh: ¾ cup
Cooked soybeans: ¾ cup
Other cooked beans: 1 cup

Cheese (firm): 2 ounces

Soft cheese (cottage cheese): ½ cup

Paneer (Indian soft cheese): ½ cup

Milk (whole or skim, or buttermilk): 1¾ cup

Yogurt: 1¾ cups

Nut butters: ¼ cup

Nuts: ½ cup

Sunflower seeds: ½ cup

Pumpkin seeds: 6 tablespoons

Whole-grain bread: 6 slices

Broccoli: 3 cups

Cooked whole grains (rice, millet, oats, quinoa, kamut, etc.): 3 cups

It is clear from the list above that vegetarians can get sufficient protein.

Below is a list[2] of nonvegetarian sources of protein:

Beef (broiled), 3 oz. = 21 to 25 grams protein

Ham (broiled), 3 oz. = 18 grams protein

Veal (broiled), 3 oz. = 23 grams protein

Chicken (roasted), 3.5 oz. = 27 grams protein

Turkey (roasted), 3.5 oz. = 28 grams protein

Salmon (baked/broiled), 3.5 oz. = 27 grams protein

Halibut (broiled), 3.5 oz. = 21 grams protein

Mackerel (broiled), 3.5 oz. = 22 grams protein

Flounder (baked), 3.5 oz. = 30 grams protein

Swordfish (broiled), 3.5 oz. = 28 grams protein

Tuna (canned in water), 3.5 oz. = 28 grams protein

Sardines (canned), 3.5 oz. = 24 grams protein

Scallops (steamed), 3.5 oz. = 18 grams protein

The larger fish (like swordfish and tuna) and shellfish, have been found to be high in mercury due to pollution. It is wise to eat these only occasionally, if at all.

Processed and cured meats, like bologna and hot dogs, are lower in protein and higher in fat. They are high in sodium and nitrates (can cause cancer). There are quality, chemical-free soy and turkey franks that are safer to eat. As a rule, avoid processed and cured meats.

Your postpartum recovery will be enhanced greatly if you've eaten sufficient protein during your pregnancy, because protein is essential for the repair and formation of new body tissue.

It is especially important to choose organic sources of protein. When pouring the foundation for a house, you would never choose poor-quality cement. Protein is the body builder. Antibodies, which fight disease, are proteins. The transportation of nutrients and oxygen through your body is dependent upon the presence of protein. All enzymes, and many of your hormones, are protein!

Many nutrition experts believe that North Americans consume more protein than they need. This may be true, but remember: pregnant women *must* eat protein. According to Anne Frye, "the nutrient needs of the pregnant woman are entirely unique . . . many of the special demands of tissue building can only be met with adequate protein . . . ."[3] Don't worry—eating adequate protein will not make your baby grow too big. In fact, the biggest baby I ever received was an 11 pounder, and his mother was a strict vegetarian.

A deeper, biochemical look at proteins reveals that they are made up of amino acids. Of the approximately twenty-nine garden-variety amino acids, eight of them are "essential." This means our bodies need them and yet we don't synthesize them ourselves. These eight amino acids must be supplied; in other words, we've got to eat them to get them. If you are an ovo-lacto vegetarian, meaning you eat eggs and dairy products, you will probably get adequate amino acids in the proper balance without much fuss. Adding poultry and/or seafoods to your diet makes it even easier.

Strict vegetarians must pay close attention to getting the essential amino acids, by combining vegetable sources of protein.

The following list[4] is a good guideline for the combining of proteins:

Rice + Legumes*
Corn + Legumes
Wheat + Legumes
Wheat + Peanuts + Milk
Wheat + Sesame + Soybeans
Rice + Nutritional yeast
Soybeans + Rice + Wheat
Soybeans + Corn + Milk
Soybeans + Wheat + Sesame
Soybeans + Peanuts + Sesame
Soybeans + Peanuts + Wheat + Rice
Sesame + Beans
Peanuts + Sunflower seeds
Lima beans, or green beans, or Brussels sprouts or cauliflower or broccoli
    + Sesame seeds or Brazil nuts or mushrooms
Millet or Rice + Greens

Note: The grains should be whole or unrefined.

(* Legumes are beans and peas. They include aduki beans, black beans, black-eyed peas, garbanzo beans, great Northern beans, kidney beans, lentils, lima beans, pinto beans, mung beans, navy beans, peanuts, soybeans, and green peas—to name a few.)

WHEN YOUR BABY CRIES FOR PROTEIN

I have found, through my own pregnancy experiences and in observing many hundreds of pregnant women in three countries, that a sure way to have a restless night is to skimp on your protein intake. If you wake up to pee (and believe me, all pregnant women wake up at night to pee), and you can't get right back to sleep, there's a reason: Your body is trying to tell you that you and the developing baby need more protein than you consumed during the day. Try eating a middle-of-the-night snack of tofu, or have some bites of chicken that you saved over from the family dinner. So far, every one of my pregnant women who has tried this trick has gone right back to sleep after satisfying the protein craving.

Also, craving sweets may mean you need protein. If your mouth is watering over chocolate chip cookies—to the point where you could easily eat half a bag of cookies—eat a tofu burger instead. Afterward, if you're really still wishing for a cookie, have one.

IRON AND PREGNANCY

Most physicians routinely prescribe an iron supplement during pregnancy. The normal hemoglobin drop that occurs during pregnancy as one's blood volume increases has caused much undue alarm. The best cure for iron deficiency, which is a precursor for anemia, is prevention. If you began your pregnancy with nutritional deficiencies, you may be more at risk for anemia. Anemia is described as, "a state characterized by deficiency of either hemoglobin or erythrocytes (blood elements which contain hemoglobin and transport oxygen) in circulating blood."[5] We will discuss good dietary sources of iron in just a bit.

You may have heard that there are "good" and "bad" kinds of iron supplements. Suffice it to say that you should never take **ferrous sulfate**. Ferrous sulfate is very hard on your liver and causes constipation. A better choice is the nonsulfate kind of iron supplement, like ferrous citrate or ferrous gluconate. Discuss this with your health-care provider if you are prescribed an iron supplement, so that you can be certain you are taking one that is beneficial.

When a pregnant woman is low in iron and/or other nutrients, she will look pale and wan. She will feel weak, run down, and have little energy. You may hear her say she feels "dull" or "brain dead." Sometimes an iron-deficient person has little or no appetite and may be constipated, which compounds the problem.

To avoid anemia in pregnancy you must assimilate iron. Low hemoglobin is also caused by the lack of many related nutrients, including copper, the B complex vitamins, protein, vitamin E, and vitamin C. Because we live in a world full of stress and environmental pollution, we need more vitamin C, which will aid in the absorption of iron. Sufficient, well-

Vegetable Sources of Iron Include[6]

+ Kale, spinach, chard, parsley, dandelion greens, beet greens, beets, apricots (if dried, soak them)
+ Prunes, raisins (soak them), prune juice
+ Whole grains (remember you can sprout grains)
+ Millet, bulgur wheat, miso, grapes
+ Blackstrap molasses, potatoes (cooked with the skin)
+ Pumpkin seeds, sesame seeds, tahini
+ Split peas, lentils, kidney beans, pinto beans, lima beans, navy beans, soybeans
+ Garbanzo beans, snap or snow peas
+ Sea vegetables, nuts, cherry juice, wheat grass juice
+ Nettle leaf, red raspberry leaf (tea or infusion)
+ Spirulina: available in powder and capsules at health food stores
+ Chlorophyll: available in both liquid and capsule form at health food stores
+ Floridex: a liquid iron supplement available at health food stores
+ Ferrum Phos: a homeopathic remedy sold at health food stores

absorbed iron in turn facilitates protein metabolism. So you see, nutrition is a wonderful gestalt.

If you are taking or plan to take an iron supplement during pregnancy, you should look to this only as "insurance." A nutritional "attitude" seeking optimal health will be the real foundation upon which you will build your iron stores. Sufficient iron (and all other nutrients) fortifies you against blood loss at the time you deliver your baby.

Foods high in iron (and copper) include seafood and meat. If you are a vegetarian, you will need to take special care to get the nutrients you need. Since most of the vegetarian women I've helped take a special interest in nutrition, I've seldom run into iron deficiencies among them. Most of these women are choosing home birth and are aware of their personal responsibility to maintain optimal health. Thus, I'm blessed to be serving a self-selected group of women who are generally in excellent health. Even in Bali and the Philippine Islands, I've found that an awareness of what constitutes good nutrition is enough to inspire even a woman with minimal resources to improve her nutrition.

Be aware that *organically* grown vegetables and grains are more abundant in iron and all vitamins and minerals. Whole, unrefined foods are also more nutritious.

Moderate exercise, such as bicycling, swimming, or walking, increases your tissue's oxygen demand and stimulates the body's effective use of iron and other nutrients. This builds better blood. To improve iron absorption, try adding a bit of citrus to your food, and remember—caffeine depletes your iron, so be mindful of your intake!

CALCIUM AND YOUR PREGNANT AND LACTATING BODY

The mineral calcium is necessary for the maintenance of your bones and teeth during pregnancy. Furthermore, it is the expectant mother who provides the calcium that, along with a medley of nutritional components, become the baby's bones. Calcium strengthens bones and teeth and helps in the transmission of nerve impulses. The proper function of one's parathyroid is maintained by calcium. This mineral is very important during pregnancy and the birth itself, as it protects the function of normal blood clotting. Calcium guards us against the effects of heavy metals and carcinogens, while balancing our blood pH[7]. It is not only important during pregnancy, but increasingly important during breastfeeding. Developing good eating habits that provide your body with enough calcium will guard you against osteoporosis later in life.

Leg cramps are a sign that your body needs additional calcium and B vitamins. Drinking milk and eating dairy products is a sure way to increase your calcium intake. There are many women who do not digest dairy products well; I found this to be especially true in Asia. There are many vegetable sources of calcium as well (see chart). When choosing a calcium supplement, the most easily assimilated form is calcium citrate maleate. Also available and effective for most women is calcium citrate and calcium carbonate. Women who are calcium-deficient suffer a decreased tolerance for pain.

Food Sources of Calcium

- Dark leafy greens, okra, broccoli, acorn squash
- Peanuts, legumes
- Milk, buttermilk, yogurt, kefir, cheese, cottage cheese
- Blackstrap molasses

The mineral magnesium and vitamin C aid your body in the assimilation of calcium.

FOLACIN

Folacin is also called folic acid. It is necessary for growth, the healthy division of cells, transference of genetic information, and the formation of red blood cells. So basic is the role of folacin that deficiencies in pregnancy can cause neural tube defects in the baby.

To get plenty of folacin, think foliage. One cup of organic, dark leafy greens (do not overcook) will provide you with one-quarter your daily requirement of folic acid during pregnancy. It is recommended that pregnant women get twice as much (800 micrograms daily) as nonpregnant women (400 micrograms daily). Look to liver, leafy greens, nuts, green beans, asparagus, legumes, lima beans, whole grains, and oranges as food sources for folacin. Good-quality vitamins, formulated for pregnancy, contain folic acid as well.

VITAMIN AND MINERAL SUPPLEMENTS

In a perfect world, all of our nutritional needs would be met from the wholesome food we eat. Unhealthy farming practices, like spraying with herbicides, fungicides, insecticides and using chemical fertilizers, have robbed our soil, and thus our food, of nutrients. Therefore, I suggest that women choose a healthy, quality vitamin and mineral supplement from natural sources formulated for pregnancy, and take it daily, as directed. Consult your midwife or physician about vitamin/mineral supplements before you begin. S/he may have an excellent recommendation regarding a quality product and advice on precautions. Despite the supplements, seek to fill your most basic nutritional needs via your food. Taking a good vitamin and eating junk does not cut it. Eat well—as well as you possibly can—and take the best pregnancy vitamin/mineral supplement that you can find.

After you have had your baby, continue to take your prenatal vitamins, at least for as long as you are breastfeeding.

COPING WITH THE DISCOMFORTS OF PREGNANCY

NAUSEA

Nausea or "morning sickness" is probably the most common pregnancy discomfort, especially in the first trimester. I wonder why it ever got called morning sickness; I had it all day during my third pregnancy.

It can range from a queasy feeling to vomiting many times a day. Poor nutrition makes the nausea associated with pregnancy worse. However, the condition itself makes it difficult to eat and often makes it difficult to keep down the food you do eat. Making every bite count, meaning eating wholesome foods, is important when you are experiencing nausea.

Most commonly, the cause of nausea is hypoglycemia (inadequate blood sugar levels). In this case the villain is often white flour, white sugar, processed foods, and poor nutrition. I hate to tell you this, but poor eating habits do make you suffer. Your organs, the pancreas in particular, strive to keep your blood sugar in balance. The stress of refined carbohydrates (foods made with white flour and sugar) cause the pancreas to release too much insulin as it tries to bring your body's glucose levels back to normal. This overreaction to simple sugars by the pancreas causes the blood sugar to drop too low. In a nutshell, this is hypoglycemia. If you crave sweets, do not cave in and eat sugar treats. They only stress your body, which is craving sugar because it needs more real nutrients.

Sometimes nausea is caused by toxic fumes or other pollutants in your environment. Be careful to avoid these.

If the nausea becomes very severe—for example you are vomiting nearly all of your food and getting dehydrated—you may have hyperemesis gravidarum. This is potentially dangerous for both you and the baby. Please see your healthcare provider so s/he can help you.

Nausea Busters

+ Many small meals throughout the day and a snack at night
+ Ginger root tea
+ Wild yam root tincture (½ dropper 2 times per day)
+ Red raspberry leaf tea
+ Peppermint or spearmint tea
+ High-protein snacks, such as bits of chicken, hard-boiled eggs, tofu, plain yogurt, cheese
+ Fresh fruit
+ Sweet potatoes

Heartburn Busters

- Avoid spicy foods
- Drink the water from a young (green) coconut
- Take a leisurely walk after meals (do not lie down)
- Sip warm milk or have a tablespoon of cream
- Avoid drinking and eating at the same time
- Chew raw nuts very well
- Sip peppermint tea
- Eat papaya or take papaya enzymes
- Try natural digestive enzyme tablets
- Eat baked potatoes, yams, and sweet potatoes—plain with a pinch of salt
- Avoid caffeine and alcohol—they stimulate excess acid
- Eat smaller meals, more frequently

HEARTBURN

Heartburn in the third trimester is not an uncommon complaint. It is caused by the hormones of pregnancy, which relax your body's soft tissues as you prepare for birth and allow the muscle separating the esophagus from your stomach to relax too much. In addition, the pressure of the baby forces small amounts of your stomach contents back up into the lower part of the esophagus. So you have partially digested food and digestive acids backing up and burning. It feels just exactly like what it is. I often tell pregnant women, "The cure is to wait it out and have your baby." On the practical side, there are a few tricks that have helped many expectant women overcome heartburn. See the box alongside.

SWELLING

Swelling of the ankles, and/or fingers, and wrists usually occurs when a pregnant woman is losing salt from perspiring, and needs more. Too much salt is not good. Too little is also not good. It is wise to salt to taste, and taste your salt. This means if you are in the habit of putting excessive amounts of salt on your food, you need to back off a little, center yourself while eating, and really enjoy the flavor of your food. When you do this, you will learn to recognize intuitively how much salt your body needs.

I tell my pregnant women to notice any early signs of swelling. Interpret this as a message from your body that says, "Take better care of me." At the first sign of swelling, drink more pure water. Pay better attention to your dietary choices. Eat wholesome organic foods, remembering to get at least two to three servings of protein daily. And, salt your food to taste. Usually this resolves the swelling within a few days.

If you have persistent swelling, called edema, you must see your health-care provider. Persistent edema is often a sign of poor nutrition, which may develop into toxemia, a potentially dangerous pregnancy complication.

CONSTIPATION

Constipation is a problem for many women during pregnancy. This is a natural reaction to hormones that prevent miscarriage. Some of my pregnant women have found that they were more constipated when they took their supplements. This is easily solved by making a habit of taking your morning prenatal vitamin/mineral supplement right after your daily bowel movement. This will give the body plenty of time to assimilate the supplement before it's again time to have a bowel movement.

Insufficient intake of fluids definitely causes constipation due to dehydration. If you can't "go," drink a tall glass of water and generally increase your liquid intake.

Remember: whole unrefined foods are less constipating as they contain more roughage.

CHANGES IN PREGNANCY

Pregnancy brings with it so many changes. Some of the changes are wonderful, others uncomfortable. Your breasts most likely will get bigger, and become tender and tingly. Your skin may glow, and any problems you've had with your complexion may clear up during pregnancy. Your hair may become thicker, shinier. Your body will gain weight. You may not wish to make love, or you may enjoy love-making even more than before. You may get some stretch marks, your

> *W*here would all the specialists and producers of medical technology and drugs be if it were suddenly 'discovered' that when women eat well in pregnancy, eliminate drugs and stop substance abuse, almost all complications disappear?"
>
> —ANNE FRYE, author of *Understanding Diagnostic Tests in the Childbearing Year and Holistic Midwifery*

back may ache some days, and your energy will fade one day and be tremendous the next. All in all, you will enjoy your pregnancy (and postpartum) more if you are well nourished. Nutrition is really a valuable tool for maintaining a healthy pregnancy. It will fortify you for the birth of your baby. A well-nourished mom feels better postpartum, and breastfeeding is more easily established. A healthy mother equals a healthy, alert, happy baby.

---

[1] Laurel Robertson, Carol Flinders and Brian Ruppenthal, *The New Laurel's Kitchen* (Berkeley, Ca.: Ten Speed Press, 1986), 369.

[2] Stanley Gershoff, Ph.D., *The Tufts University Guide to Total Nutrition* (New York: Harper and Row, 1990), 10.

[3] Anne Frye, *Holistic Midwifery Volume I* (Portland, Ore.: Labrys Press, 1998), 219.

[4] Ibid.

[5] *Dorland's Pocket Medical Dictionary 21st edition* (Philadelphia, London, Toronto: W.B. Saunders Co. 1968), 31.

[6] Robin Lim, *After the Baby's Birth* (Berkeley, Ca.: Celestial Arts, 2001), 186 -187.
Laurel Robertson, Carol Flinders and Brian Ruppenthal, *The New Laurel's Kitchen* (Berkeley, Ca.: Ten Speed Press, 1986), 370.
Elison M. Hass, M.D., *Staying Healthy with Nutrition* (Berkeley, Ca.: Celestial Arts, 1992), 333.
Ina May Gaskin, *Spiritual Midwifery, Third Edition* (Summertown, Tenn.: The Book Publishing Co., 1990), 222.
Anne Frye, *Holistic Midwifery Volume I* (Portland Ore.: Labrys Press, 1998), 134-136 .

[7] Anne Frye, *Holistic Midwifery Volume I* (Portland Ore.: Labrys Press, 1998), 224.

What to Avoid During Pregnancy

For the health and well-being of your baby, and for yourself, absolutely avoid alcohol, cigarettes, and all drugs. Following is a guide to help pregnant and breastfeeding women avoid substances and circumstances that may be harmful to a developing or breastfed baby. Regarding all artificial substances: *when in doubt, leave it out.* All mothers worry, "Will my baby be all right?" The best we can do during pregnancy is to avoid potentially dangerous situations, think positive thoughts, and offer up our fears to a Higher Power. Please try not to worry too much, as excessive worrying can also be harmful to you and your baby.

SMOKING

Cigarette smoking (and marijuana smoking) reduces blood flow to the placenta; this does cause the baby to suffer. Clearly, smoking is linked to decreased birth weight, which increases the risk of miscarriage and stillbirth.[1] The more one smokes, the greater the risk of miscarriage, problems with the placenta, premature rupture of membranes, and even fetal and newborn death. Once the baby is born, s/he is still not out of the woods; maternal smoking during pregnancy may have long-term effects on the child's growth and intellectual development. Children who grow up with parents who smoke suffer more respiratory illnesses and infections, and they are at increased risk for childhood cancer.

Cigarette smoke contains 68,000 toxic substances.[2] Now is the time to quit smoking. It is an addiction, and though it is a hard habit to break, it can be done. Many, many women have quit smoking during pregnancy. For these women and their babies, the benefits are immediate: Within forty-eight hours after a pregnant woman stops smoking, her blood carries eight percent more oxygen to her baby![3]

ALCOHOL

Alcohol, which is ethanol, and is found in hard liquor, beer, and wine, increases the risk of miscarriage. It can cause Fetal Alcohol Syndrome

(FAS), which itself manifests in physical abnormalities of the head and face and in abnormalities of the brain and central nervous system of the child. FAS manifestations may include the most serious alcohol-related birth defect: retardation. It is estimated that 30 to 40 percent of the off-spring of alcoholic mothers are expected to show the complete syndrome.[4]

Alcohol can also cause Fetal Alcohol Effect (FAE), resulting in any number of problems, including eye and heart defects; lung, kidney and other organ impairment; slowed growth; irritability; behavioral problems; and neuromuscular defects.[5] Alcohol is also known to cause low birth weight, the precursor for all kinds of problems, including increased incidence of infant mortality.

Even an occasional drink is not worth the risks. There is no known safe, minimal amount of alcohol consumption. Just don't do it. Women who have consumed some alcohol during pregnancy should know that stopping benefits the baby immediately.

CAFFEINE

Caffeine is a stimulant and a stressor. It crosses the placenta and affects the baby. Because the fetal liver cannot process caffeine as quickly as the mother's, it stays in the baby's bloodstream for a long time.

Caffeine is found in coffee, instant coffee, black tea, chocolate, cocoa drinks, some over-the-counter medications (read the label and consult your health-care provider), and some soft drinks and sodas. There are now many soft drinks available that are caffeine free; some are even made with organic ingredients (read the label). It is wiser, however, to choose to drink good old H_2O, and plenty of it.

Caffeine should be eliminated during pregnancy. It also crosses into breast milk, and should not be ingested by nursing mothers. Commonly, caffeine causes anxiety, restlessness, diarrhea, headaches, and heartburn. You may feel more alert on caffeine, yet it impairs your fine-motor coordination. Too much caffeine can cause insomnia, tremors, and ringing in the ears. A little may be too much, depending upon the individual. It stresses the adrenal glands and impairs the immune system. Many people experience chronic fatigue and illness as a result. Since it affects the smooth cardiac muscles, caffeine can cause one's heart to beat irregularly. Breast lumps have been directly related to the ingestion of caffeine.

To quit caffeine, make the decision and stick by it. You can drink herbal teas (see Herbs to Avoid During Pregnancy, page 36) or grain-based coffee substitutes instead. Some of these are delicious and soothing. Often, coffee is decaffeinated using a harsh chemical process. You can find coffee that is decaffeinated using the Swiss water process. Pregnant women (and everybody) should choose this over the chemically decaffeinated variety.

I admit to having had a period in my life when I was addicted to coffee. I woke up one morning and realized that I was, most likely, newly pregnant (this would be my third baby). So I quit drinking coffee, cold turkey. It took a lot of resolve, as I had headaches and the worst nausea I had ever experienced. My midwife advised me to drink more water and get more rest. This really helped relieve my symptoms. I still adore the smell of freshly brewed coffee, but because coming off of it made me so sick, I still am afraid to drink it, seventeen years later. My baby, a girl we named Zhòu, is lovely: she just finished her home-schooling high school curriculum and is choosing a college as I write this.

Drinking alcohol, smoking cigarettes, and ingesting caffeine all too often go hand in hand. Honestly, if you avoid these harmful substances, your baby will be healthier, smarter, more alert, and yet more tranquil. It is a sacrifice worth making.

FOODS TO AVOID

Never eat even slightly spoiled food. Clean your refrigerator regularly, and make sure your refrigerator is at 40° F or below.

Undercooked or raw meats can contain parasites and are a breeding ground for dangerous bacteria. (Sorry, no sashimi while you're pregnant.) Undercooked or raw meats and fish pose a threat to pregnancy. They must be avoided. Some commercial meats contain hormones; to be safe, choose organic.

Hot dogs, luncheon or deli meats, pâté, refrigerated smoked seafood, and soft cheeses, such as Brie, Camembert, blue cheese, and queso blanco de fresco (Mexican-style fresh cheese) put pregnant and breastfeeding women at risk for listeriosis, the harmful bacteria caused by *Listeria monocytogenes.* The Center for Disease Control says that an estimated 2,500 people become seriously ill with listeriosis each year. Hormonal changes during pregnancy have an effect on your immune system that cause an increased susceptibility to listeriosis. Listeriosis can be transmitted to the developing baby through the placenta, even if the mother is not showing signs of illness. This can lead to miscarriage, premature delivery, serious health problems for the baby, and even stillbirth. To avoid this serious threat to pregnancy, avoid the foods listed above.

Trans-fatty acids, or TFAs, are unnatural forms of fatty acids. Mothers should be warned that trans-fatty acids pose a significant risk to human health. TFAs are bad for hearts and arteries and have been found to have ill effects on membrane and hormone function. According to Andrew Weil, M.D., they (TFAs) promote the development of cancer and degenerative disease, increase inflammation, accelerate aging, and obstruct immunity and healing."[6]

Partially hydrogenated oils (including partially hydrogenated soybean oil, cottonseed oil, soybean and/or corn oil) are full of TFAs. If you read the labels you will find these unhealthy oils in many, many packaged foods from the supermarket. Cookies, crackers, pastries, snack foods, and chips are among the products made with oils containing TFAs. They should be avoided, yet they are marketed aggressively as foods for children!

Margarine has as high as 30 to 40 percent TFAs and should also be avoided along with vegetable shortening, and all products made with either. In 1999 the Food and Drug Administration began requiring that food labels list include trans-fatty acids.

Olive oil is a healthy alternative. Especially extra virgin olive oil, which is gently pressed, without using harsh methods. Excellent sources of omega-3 fatty acids, which is essential to our health, are flaxseed oil and hemp oil, both healthy choices. When heating oil, avoid allowing it to smoke, as the nutritional value will be lost. Once opened, oil (other than olive oil) should be stored in the refrigerator.

PRESCRIPTION DRUGS AND NATURAL REMEDIES

If your doctor prescribes a medication, make sure s/he knows full well that you are pregnant or breastfeeding. Don't be shy to question your physician about the possible side effects of medications; s/he will appreciate your concern. You may ask to look up prescribed drugs in the book *Drugs in Pregnancy and Lactation . . . A Reference Guide to Fetal and Neonatal Risk,* by Gerald G. Briggs, Roger K. Freeman, and Sumner J. Yaffe. Also, get another opinion if you have any doubts about prescription or over-the-counter drugs. Even aspirin and acne medications (such as Acutane) should be avoided. Birth control pills should be discontinued immediately if pregnancy is suspected.

Laxatives (even natural or herbal laxatives, such as flaxseed, senna, aloe, castor oil, turkey rhubarb, buckthorn, and cascare sagrada) should be avoided.

Do not dye your hair while you are pregnant. Prolonged exposure to extremely high temperatures (such as in hot tubs) also poses a risk.

Read the ingredients when you are choosing a commercial herbal tea. There are many herbs that are beneficial during pregnancy and lactation, but some should be avoided (see box, page 36). Some herbal preparations made especially for pregnant women may contain some of the herbs to avoid. Consult your midwife or doctor before taking any of these products.

FASTING

Pregnant and breastfeeding women should never fast. Please, don't try it. Fasting during pregnancy will compromise your health and that of your baby.

It is, however, very wise to drink the pure, freshly made juice of apples, pears, and beets, which cleanse the liver and are full of nutrients. Also drink, daily if possible, the pure, fresh juice of oranges, which will enliven you with vitamin C.

Herbs to Avoid During Pregnancy

Angelica	Licorice root
Aloe leaves	Liferoot
Bethroot	Lobelia
Birthroot	Lovage root
Black cohosh root	Marijuana
Blue cohosh root	Mistletoe
Catnip	Motherwort
Cotton root bark	Mugwort
Devil's claw	Osha root
Ephedra nevadenis (Mormon tea)	Papaya leaves
	Pennyroyal
Ephedra virdis (Squaw tea)	Peruvian bark
European vervain	Rue
Ergot fungus	Saffron
Feverfew	Senna
Hydrangea	Shave grass (horsetail)
Hyssop	
Jimsonweed	Tansy
Juniper	Wormwood

ENVIRONMENTAL POLLUTANTS

Avoid environmental pollutants such as pesticides, herbicides, and fungicides; and heavy metals such as lead, nickel, cadmium, and manganese, for your safety and the baby's health. Even car exhaust should be avoided.

TOXIC HOUSEHOLD SUBSTANCES

Look around your home. You may find many poisons and harmful substances that you must not use while pregnant or breastfeeding. These include turpentine, paint thinner, oven cleaners, lacquer thinner, dry-cleaning fluids, oil-based paints, stains, contact cement, model-airplane glue, fiberglass emulsion, bug sprays, nail polish remover, and hairspray.

CAT AND BIRD FECES

Cat and bird feces can contain toxoplasmosis, a harmful organism. If you have a cat that uses a liter box, you should never be the one to empty or clean it while you are pregnant. Nor should you handle bird droppings. Maternal infection from toxoplasmosis can cause damage to the baby.

X RAYS AND ELECTROMAGNETIC FIELDS

Avoid **diagnostic X rays.** Let your doctor or dentist know you are pregnant. Do not assume s/he knows, even if you've mentioned it previously. If there is no alternative to the X ray, ask for extra protective covering.

There is evidence that **electromagnetic fields** are harmful. In my own midwifery practice, I've noticed that in a specific area of housing that has a strong electromagnetic field, many miscarriages have occurred. Do not spend time in places you suspect have strong electromagnetic fields, like power stations and places where there are a lot of live electrical cables.

---

1 Gerald G. Briggs, Roger K. Freeman, Sumner J. Yaffe, *Drugs in Pregnancy and Lactation 4th Edition* (Baltimore, Md.:,1994), 343 and Council on Scientific Affairs, American Medical Assn. "Fetal Effects of Maternal Alcohol." *JAMA* 1983;249:2517-21.

2 Anne Frye, *Holistic Midwifery Volume I* (Portland Ore.:, Labrys Press, 1998), 275.

3 Ibid., 266-69, and Laurel Robertson, Carol Flinders and Brian Ruppenthal, *The New Laurel's Kitchen* (Berkeley, Ca.: Ten Speed Press, 1986), 372.

4 Anne Frye, *Holistic Midwifery Volume I* (Portland Ore.:, Labrys Press, 1998), 266.

5 Ibid., 269

6 Andrew Weil, M.D., *Eating Well for Optimal Health* (New York: Alfred A. Knopf, 2000), 93.

Genetically Engineered Foods...
Are They Safe?

A new page in history has been turned. Scientists can now change the DNA of living organisms; this is what genetic engineering is.

DNA is the blueprint for every life-form. Life itself, growth, and every unique feature, function, and biochemical process of individual organisms is dependent upon its specific DNA.

Using enzymes to cut and splice specific gene segments from the DNA of living organisms, molecular biologists can now customize food plants. Vectors—strands of DNA (such as viruses that infect cells and insert themselves into DNA)—can be used to build new living organisms never before seen on Earth. The harvest and products of these organisms has never before been a part of the human food supply.

Genetic engineers believe that this technique will improve the foods we eat. For example, scientists used this technology to insert a gene from the flounder fish, which resists the cold, into tomato DNA. The results are tomatoes that are resistant to frost and have a longer growing season. Exciting? Yes. Yet, we must ask the next question: Are these man-made organisms, which now carry the gene of an animal, still plants?

And the next question: What are the long-term effects on humans, and other animals, when they ingest the fruit, root, or seeds of genetically engineered organisms?

Sadly, in fact dangerously, foods from these customized organisms are already on the market, and there has not been time for long-term rigorous research and testing. The long-term effects of genetically modified foods on our health and our environment are virtually unknown.

Genetic engineering can cause organisms to mutate, which can create new and higher levels of toxins in foods. Genetically engineered foods can create new and unforeseen allergens in foods.

Since genetically engineered crops contain genes that confer resistance to antibiotics, what will happen if these antibiotic-resistant genes are assimilated by bacteria that can infect us?

In a series of experiments in which pregnant mice were fed the DNA of bacteriophage M13, fragments of the DNA survived passage through the gastrointestinal tract of the mother mice in small amounts (1 to 2 percent). Later, this M13 DNA was detected in the cells of various organs of the mouse fetuses and newborns (not in all their cells). This means there is evidence to assume that food-ingested foreign DNA can become covalently linked to mouse DNA.[1]

And the next question is.... Can this happen to humans? So far the only answers we have are: We don't know, and maybe.

To be safe, all people, especially pregnant women, should try to avoid genetically engineered or genetically modified foods. The following is a list of genetically engineered crops that have already been approved for sale:

- canola
- corn (including popcorn and sweet corn, not blue corn)
- cotton
- flax
- papaya
- potatoes (Burbank Russet)
- soybeans
- yellow crookneck squash
- sugar beets
- tomatoes (including cherry)

Fortunately, consumer concerns have caused the larger buyers of potatoes to favor genetically natural potatoes, so GE potato planting is on the decline.

The latest reports on the Mothers for Natural Law web site are that GE tomatoes are no longer on the market.

Though GE flax was approved for release, the Flax Council of Canada successfully petitioned against planting it. The GE seed was crushed, all 600,000 bushels of it, and in this way kept out of our food supply.

Mothers should note that the list of foods to be careful about include dairy products from cows injected with recombinant bovine growth hormone (rGBH is a hormone produced by genetically modified organisms). Check the label; make sure to buy only rGBH-free milk, butter, yogurt, cheese, cream, buttermilk, and whey.

Animal feed often contains genetically engineered organisms. Be suspicious of all animal products (and by-products), such as meat and dairy.

Vegetable oils containing corn, soybeans, canola, and cotton should be avoided. Olive oil is a safer choice.

Be careful when choosing packaged and processed foods. Read the labels. If it mentions any of the ingredients in the list above, without specifying it as organic, then the product probably contains genetically engineered ingredients. Better yet, choose against packaged and processed food.

Because GE soybeans have been used in infant formula, breastfeeding is even more important today than in the past. The best way to protect your baby from GE foods is to breastfeed.

To avoid the potential dangers of genetically engineered foods, choose to buy, grow, and eat fresh organic produce. For your family's protection, choose organic meat and dairy products.

As mothers we are voting every day, at the cash register. If we refuse to buy GE foods to feed our families, we are discouraging the use of this potentially dangerous technology. In this way we protect our families, our environment, and our future food supply.

For more detailed information please visit the Mothers for Natural Law web site at www.safe-food.org.

1 Shubbert, R., et al., 1998. Ingested foreign (phage M13) DNA survives transiently in the gastrointestinal tract and enter the bloodstream of mice. *Mol. Gen. Genet* 242: 495-504.

and

Doerfler, W., and Schubbert, R., 1998. Uptake of foreign DNA from the environment: the gastrointestinal tract and the placenta as portals of entry. *Wein Klin Worchenschr,* 110 (2) : 40-4.

Found on:

The Mothers for Natural Law web site http://www.safe-food.org

About Eggs

*M*any breakfast dishes are made with eggs. Eggs are a concentrated food source, so it's important to choose organic. This means the hens are fed organic food, with no additives. "Free-range" is best, because the chickens are allowed to run around in the fresh air and sunshine. Organic free-range eggs are more expensive than eggs laid by chickens raised in closed quarters and fed grain loaded with hormones, stimulants, and antibiotics, but they're well worth it. When one considers the protein content of an egg, it's a miracle food and a bargain at any price. When we are in the United States, our family stays in Iowa. Mr. Williams, a local farmer, delivers eggs to our kitchen from hens his wife pampers and feeds with grain grown in their own fields.

Besides being 50 percent protein, eggs contain all the essential amino acids our bodies need. Eggs have taken a bad rap for containing fat and cholesterol. Recently research has shown that if you do not partake of a high-fat diet, eggs will not raise your serum cholesterol. Translation: Avoid the bacon or sausage, and partake in organic eggs, without overdoing the butter. If you have a history of cardiovascular disease or high cholesterol, eggs should be avoided.

The yolk contains 3 grams of protein, is quite high in vitamin A and B vitamins, vitamins D and E, calcium, iron, phosphorus, zinc, and selenium. Egg whites contain protein, fewer calories than the yolk, some selenium, no fat, and also no vitamin A.

BREAKFAST

Pregnant women need between 100 and 400 calories more per day than nonpregnant women. A lactating mother needs 500 additional calories daily. From bedtime to breakfast is a long stretch: You will find that if you delay or skip breakfast, you can feel impaired all day.

In the first trimester many women are plagued with nausea. One of the best remedies for pregnancy nausea is to eat something nourishing immediately upon rising. At our house, my husband, Wil, better know as "Dad," "Lolo" (grandpa in Tagalog), or "BaPak" (father in Bahasa Indonesia) is the breakfast chef. Upon rising my granddaughter will often appear at our bedside and say "Lolo, I'm es-tremely hungry." Many of these rise-and-shine recipes are inspired by and invented by him.

Scrambled Tofu

SERVES 4 TO 6

1 tablespoon toasted sesame oil

1 tablespoon extra virgin olive oil

1/4 teaspoon cumin seeds

1/2 medium yellow onion, diced (optional)

2 pounds firm tofu, crumbled

1 green or red bell pepper, seeded and diced

1/2 teaspoon ground turmeric

Salt

1 cup grated Jack or cheddar cheese (optional)

Tofu contains some protein as well as calcium, iron, and phosphorus. Serve with whole-grain toast or Garlic Rice (page 53).

In a large cast-iron skillet or wok, heat the oils over low heat and gently brown cumin seeds. Add the onion and sauté until translucent. Add the tofu, pepper, and turmeric, and salt to taste. Mix, cover, and cook over low heat for 10 to 15 minutes. If you choose to add cheese, sprinkle it over the tofu in the last 3 minutes of cooking, and replace the cover until the cheese is melted. Serve hot.

Bull's Eye

SERVES 1

This breakfast recipe has become a family tradition at our house. Our children introduced it to their friends in Bali, and now it's a village favorite, too.

Using a cup or jar, cut a round hole in the center of the slice of bread. Pour a thin coating of oil into a cast-iron skillet over medium heat. When oil is hot, drop the bread in, and break the egg into the hole. Fit the center of the bread alongside the egg/bread. When the white looks nearly done, flip it. Also flip the bread circle. When the white appears well done and the yellow of the egg is done to the specification of the eater, serve it up with paprika and pepper to taste. Some people in our family prefer "over easy," and others want their eggs "over hard," so we cook their eggs longer. Serve immediately.

I slice whole-grain bread

Extra virgin olive oil

I large egg

Paprika and/or freshly ground black pepper (optional)

Perfect Boiled Eggs

To make perfect soft-boiled, medium-cooked, or hard-boiled eggs, follow these simple directions. The method is the same for both soft and hard-boiled eggs; only the timing is different. For breakfast, enjoy your eggs with a slice of whole-grain toast.

Place eggs in a saucepan. Cover them with cold water. Cook over medium heat, bringing the water to the boiling point. Lower the heat to a simmer.

Watch the time.

For soft-boiled eggs, cook 2 to 3 minutes (3 to 4 if eggs were cold from refrigerator). For **medium-cooked eggs,** cook about 4 minutes (add about a minute for cold eggs). For **hard-boiled eggs,** cook 10 to 15 minutes. (If you are doing many eggs at once the cooking time is a little longer.) To prevent discoloration of the yolks, run cold water over hard-boiled eggs immediately after removing them from the heat.

To open and serve a soft-boiled egg, use a butter knife: gently tap around the center, breaking the shell and then cutting the egg in half. Be careful not to create too many bits of shell; these must not get into the egg. Once the soft-boiled egg is split open, scoop it into a tea cup. Medium-cooked eggs will open the same way, but are less sloppy, so they are easier to manage. Add a bit of salt and pepper, and enjoy.

To peel hard-boiled eggs, tap the egg to crack the shell. Roll the egg in your hands to free the shell from the interior tough skin. Don't be annoyed if your hard-boiled egg is difficult to peel; it means the egg is very, very fresh.

Cresencia's Deviled Eggs

SERVES 4 TO 6

I include this recipe in the breakfast section to keep it close to the instructions for perfect boiled eggs. Personally, I like to eat deviled eggs for breakfast. Make deviled eggs ahead and save a couple for your middle-of-the-night high-protein snack. This version is what I grew up on; it was served by my mother, Cresencia Lim Jehle.

Slice the eggs in half, lengthwise. Carefully remove yolks without damaging the whites. Crush the yolks gently with a fork, mixing with the mayonnaise to moisten. Add the mustard, paprika, and chives. Salt to taste. Spoon the filling back into the egg white halves, garnish with the olive slices, mint, rosemary, or capers, and serve.

4 to 6 hard-boiled eggs (see page 46), shelled

2 tablespoons mayonnaise or sour cream

I teaspoon Dijon mustard

Pinch sweet paprika

¼ cup chopped fresh chives (optional)

Sea salt

Olive slices, fresh mint or rosemary sprigs, or capers, for garnish

4 to 6 large eggs

Pinch of sweet paprika

2 tablespoons soy milk or filtered water

Sea salt

Extra virgin olive oil

1 medium onion, diced

A generous handful of finely chopped kale leaves

1 large green bell pepper, seeded and diced

¾ cup grated Swiss cheese, (optional)

Green Pepper Omelet

SERVES 4

Some mornings "Lolo" makes short-order breakfasts, and everyone puts in a request. When we have a tighter schedule, Wil greets the morning with a steaming family-size omelet and a hill of whole-grain toast. He rounds it off with Papaya-Banana Morning Salad (see page 57) and warm chai. It's so pleasurable to eat his omelet that it's difficult to leave.

Vigorously mix the eggs, paprika, and soy milk in a medium bowl; season with salt. Heat a thin coating of oil in a large cast-iron skillet over low heat. Toss in the onion, kale, and green pepper. Stir-fry until vegetables are just barely tender, about 1 minute. Stir in the scrambled eggs and stir until the eggs set, about 3 minutes. Lower the heat, sprinkle in the Swiss cheese, and cover. Let this steam for a couple of minutes, then serve.

Becca's Breakfast Frittata

SERVES 4

An invention from Rebecca, mom of Surreal and Inti, devoted wife of Scott (better known as Tito). Best if served while singing. For the vegetables that go into the frittata, Becca says to go shopping in your fridge and see what you have. Serve immediately with steaming cups of tea and fruit on the side.

Preheat the oven to 350° F. Cut the vegetables into bite-sized pieces.

In a large cast-iron skillet with an oven-proof handle and a lid, warm the oil over medium-high heat. Add the onions and garlic and sauté. Add the vegetables that take longer to cook, like potatoes, broccoli, cauliflower, and carrots. Sauté them for 1 to 2 minutes; cover for 1 to 2 minutes, checking them often to avoid over-cooking. Next add the quicker-cooking veggies, like bell peppers, peas, and green beans. Leafy greens should be added last. Don't worry about cooking the veggies all the way: They will bake with the eggs.

Mix the eggs, salt, pepper, paprika, and milk in a medium bowl. Pour the eggs over the sautéed vegetables and sprinkle the cheese on top. Place the skillet into the oven. Bake until the eggs are firmly set, 20 to 30 minutes. The top will be a beautiful golden brown.

Approximately 2 cups assorted vegetables, such as diced cooked white or sweet potatoes, snap peas or trimmed green beans, sliced carrots or broccoli, leafy greens or diced red bell peppers

2 tablespoons extra virgin olive oil

1 small onion, diced

1 to 2 cloves garlic, minced (optional)

8 large eggs, beaten

Pinch of sea salt, pinch of freshly ground black pepper

Pinch of paprika

½ cup soy milk or cow's milk

¾ cup grated cheddar cheese or crumbled feta

2 to 4 cups filtered water, depending upon the kind of oats

1 cup oats

Butter (optional)

Ground nutmeg, ground cinnamon, or ground cardamom (optional)

Oatmeal

SERVES 4 TO 6

Research tells us that oats are healthy for the heart and cardiovascular system. Oats are 10 to 15 percent protein, and free of cholesterol and saturated fat. You can depend upon oats to provide you with some iron, magnesium, zinc, calcium, potassium, manganese, copper, folic acid, niacin, pyridoxine, and pantothenic acid. Oats are available in several thicknesses: The "quick" variety is very thin and easy to digest. It requires less water and less cooking. You can get our family favorite, "old-fashioned" or thick. We also like the chewier (nuttier-flavored) "steel-cut" oats over the rolled or flattened kind. Steel-cut oats require the most water and the longest cooking. Try steel-cut Irish oatmeal: the coarseness of the grain will surprise you, as will the deeply good flavor—though the nutritional value of oats does not suffer too much from rolling or cutting.

You may wish to add coconut to your oatmeal. Raisins and other dried fruits add nutritional value, as do chopped nuts. Fresh fruit can be added after cooking, right into each individual's bowl, or on the side. Try bananas, fresh peaches, pear, apple, papaya, mango . . . let yourself experiment. You can choose from a variety of sweeteners. Organic brown sugar is traditional. Honey is our favorite. Rice syrup or pure maple syrup are just divine.

Well-cooked oats are more digestible, so I err on the side of generous amounts of water and a longer cooking time.

Bring the water to a boil in a medium saucepan. Stir in the oats, trying to keep them from lumping. Add a dollop of butter and the spices of your choice. Decrease the heat to lowest setting and cover. Check occasionally to see if they are ready. Serve hot.

Muesli

SERVES 2 TO 4

Muesli became a favorite of mine when I was cooking in France. I was fortunate enough to be flown over to France by Maharishi International University, because they desperately needed cooks. At first I thought my European workmates were a little strange, eating this "raw" oatmeal. But once I tried it, I began to see why they were so enthusiastic about it. The overnight soaking really makes it wonderful. Try for yourself.

Combine the oats, water, salt, and spice. Let soak overnight. In the morning, add any or all of the suggested ingredients. Try serving it with milk or fruit juice.

I cup rolled or old-fashioned oats

I cup boiling filtered water

¼ teaspoon sea salt

Pinch of ground cinnamon, ground nutmeg, any spices you like

SUGGESTED ADDITIONS

Honey

Raisins

Prunes

Dried or fresh apricots

Peaches—dried or fresh

Chopped dates

Chopped nuts

Diced or grated apple, sprinkled with lemon juice

Cubed papaya

Cubed mango

Sliced bananas

Morning Rice

SERVES 4 TO 6

1 cup brown rice

4 cups filtered water

1 cinnamon stick

1 teaspoon ground cardamom

½ teaspoon ground ginger

2 cups milk

½ cup raw sugar or Sucanat

½ cup blanched almonds, coarsely ground

¼ cup raisins

¼ teaspoon sweet paprika (optional)

New mothers need something warm, nourishing, and easily digested to start their day. This is a very traditional Ayurvedic morning meal or mid-morning snack. Almonds provide protein, and can be ground in a blender. Try Morning Rice with a simple hard-boiled egg.

Grind the rice in a blender until it has the consistency of coarse sand. In a large pot, bring the water to a boil. Decrease the heat and add the cinnamon stick, cardamom, and ginger. Add the ground rice while stirring with a whisk. Simmer, uncovered, for about 30 minutes; enjoy the aroma. Stir often: don't let it stick to the bottom of the pot.

In a separate bowl, mix the milk, sugar, almonds, raisins, and paprika.

Taste the rice to make sure it is well cooked; it should have the texture of a porridge. Add the milk mixture and continue to stir. Simmer for 10 more minutes. The rice should have the consistency of thin gruel. Serve warm.

Garlic Rice

SERVES 4

Garlic rice is the national breakfast of the Philippine Islands. I remember many a sweet morning waking to the smell of my lola *(grandmother) making garlic rice. This is the perfect way to use rice left over from the night before. Use as little or as much garlic as you please.*

In a wok or large cast-iron skillet, heat a thin layer of oil over medium-low heat. Add the garlic and gently sauté it about 2 minutes until golden. Add the rice and salt to taste, mixing well. Reduce the heat to the lowest setting, cover, and let cook until the rice is evenly heated and steaming, about 15 minutes. Serve hot. *Masarap!* (Delicious!)

Extra virgin olive oil and/or toasted sesame oil

1 to 4 cloves garlic, minced

4 to 6 cups cooked rice

Sea salt

1 cup sifted whole-grain
  flour (whole wheat, spelt,
  buckwheat, etc.)

1 teaspoon natural baking
  powder

½ teaspoon sea salt

2 teaspoons raw sugar or
  Sucanat

1 large egg, beaten

1 cup milk, buttermilk, or
  plain yogurt

¼ cup butter, melted

Basic Pancakes

MAKES 6 TO 8 PANCAKES

This recipe is like an empty canvas upon which you can paint your family's favorite flavors. Enjoy with your favorite fruit and maple syrup, favorite chutney, or pesto. Remember: pancakes are not just for breakfast.

Preheat the oven to 200°F and set a stoneware plate in the oven.

Combine the flour, baking powder, salt, and sugar in a medium bowl. In a separate smaller bowl, beat together the egg, milk, and butter. Gradually add the wet ingredients to the dry ingredients, stirring only until the batter is slightly lumpy.

Oil a cast-iron skillet or griddle and heat over medium heat. Ladle the batter onto the hot skillet. Cook until you see bubbles and the edges of the pancakes appear dry. Turn only once. Keep the pancakes warm in the oven while you continue to make more pancakes.

Spicy Pancakes

Add: ¼ cup hulled, roasted pumpkin seeds and ½ teaspoon ground cumin to the dry ingredients. Add 1 tablespoon Dijon mustard and 1 to 2 tablespoons balsamic vinegar to the wet ingredients. Prepare the batter as directed above and cook as you would Basic Pancakes.

Bruce's Root Beer Pancakes

MAKES 6 TO 8 PANCAKES

Our friend Bruce is one of Earth's angels; he's always willing to help. When we were busy moving house, he surprised our family with these delightful root beer pancakes. He says they can also be made with raspberry soda, or any of your favorite carbonated drinks. Note that no baking powder is needed. Bruce serves his pancakes with finely diced parsley, sprouted sunflower seeds, and real maple syrup.

Combine the flour, salt, and sugar in a medium bowl. In a separate smaller bowl, beat together the egg, root beer, and butter. Gradually add the wet ingredients to the dry ingredients, stirring until batter is still slightly lumpy. Ladle the batter onto a very hot, oiled cast-iron skillet or griddle. Cook until you see bubbles and the edges of the pancakes appear dry. Turn only once.

1 cup sifted whole-grain flour (whole wheat, spelt, buckwheat, etc.)

½ teaspoon sea salt

2 to 3 teaspoons raw sugar or Sucanat

1 large egg, beaten

1 cup root beer

¼ cup butter, melted

OPTIONAL TOPPINGS
Sunflower or pumpkin seeds

Sesame seeds

Raisins or sliced bananas

⅓ cup quinoa flour (or substitute spelt or whole wheat flour)

⅓ cup cornmeal

⅓ cup rolled oats or rolled barley flakes

½ teaspoon sea salt

½ teaspoon natural baking soda

½ teaspoon natural baking powder

1 cup apple juice, orange juice, or buttermilk

2 tablespoons sunflower oil

2 large eggs

Wholesome Pancakes

MAKES 8 PANCAKES

Leave it to Megan, the beautiful and multitalented mother of Corwin, to have a wholesome and flavorful recipe for whole-grain pancakes. Serve with real maple syrup and fresh fruit. My children also like to put a dollop of yogurt on top. This recipe doubles nicely.

Stir together all the dry ingredients. In a separate bowl, whisk together the juice, oil, and eggs. Add the wet ingredients to the dry ingredients and mix well.

Ladle the batter on an oiled cast-iron griddle. Cook until bubbles appear, and turn. Serve hot.

Can't Sleep?

*P*regnant women often tell me that they awaken in the night and can't get back to sleep. The best solution is to eat a midnight snack packed with protein! You'll find that if you give your body what it needs, you can get right back to sleep. I recommend the following high-protein foods be kept on hand:

Grilled or roasted chicken: bite-size chunks

Tofu: cut into cubes and sprinkled with soy sauce

Hard-boiled eggs

Handful of nuts (chew well)

Nut-butter sandwich on whole-grain bread

Warm cup of milk (soy, rice, goat, or cow's milk)

Papaya-Banana Morning Salad

SERVES 4 TO 6

This wake-up salad will help aid your digestion. The bananas contain iron, magnesium, potassium, and selenium. Eat them ripe, as they will be easier to digest that way. Papayas provide beta-carotene, and are also rich in vitamin C, potassium, and minerals. The enzyme papain in papayas supports digestion. Just look at the color of this lovely fruit: It jumps up and sings! The lime is rejuvenating, purifying, detoxifying, and full of vitamins.

Toss the papaya, banana, lime juice, and coconut together in a serving bowl. Enjoy the smiles.

I medium papaya, peeled and cut into bite-size pieces

2 bananas, sliced into bite-size rounds

Squeeze of lime or lemon (optional)

$\frac{1}{4}$ cup dried shredded coconut

7 large baking potatoes (you can substitute sweet potatoes) or 10 medium potatoes, cubed

3 to 4 tablespoons extra-virgin olive oil

Generous handful fresh garden herbs, such as basil, mint, rosemary, oregano, thyme, sage, parsley, tarragon, or garlic chives, minced, or 1 tablespoon dried

Sea salt

Tomatoes, sliced (optional)

Cucumbers, diced (optional)

Cu-Cu's Hash-Browned Potatoes

SERVES 6

I named this dish after my granddaughter, Zhòuie, whom we call "Cu-Cu," which means grandchild in Bahasa Indonesia. She loves hash-browned potatoes. This goes well with eggs, cooked your favorite way.

Boil the potatoes in water to cover until they are just barely done, about 4 to 5 minutes. Drain and pat dry. In a large cast-iron skillet, heat the olive oil over medium heat (do not let it smoke or burn). If you are using dried herbs, sauté them momentarily in the warming oil. Add the potatoes and stir occasionally as the bottoms begin to brown. If you are using fresh herbs, sprinkle over the potatoes as they brown. Keep turning the potatoes until they become golden brown. Add salt to taste. If you have ripe tomatoes in your garden, slice them and serve with the hash browned potatoes. Diced cucumbers also go nicely.

FRUITS AND BEVERAGES

*T*he importance of fruit cannot be overstated. Pregnant and breastfeeding women really do benefit from the vitamin C found abundantly in fruit. Our bodies also need bioflavonoids, also known as vitamin P. Bioflavonoids are usually found in the same foods as vitamin C, which is why natural forms of vitamin C, like fruit, are more effective than synthetic ascorbic acid. Translation: Taking a pill is not as beneficial as eating a peach, tangerine, or mango. To prevent or decrease varicose veins and swelling, also known as edema, eat your fruit!

Rujak • Fruit Salad • Banana Raita • Pear Salad • Simple Papaya
Lychee Nut Balls • Almond-Banana Smoothie
Alesia's Life-Saving Date Shake • Aam or Mango Lassi
Summertime Smoothie • Sammy's Silken Tofu Smoothie
Avocado-Kiwi Cooler • Caffeine-Free Chai • Lemon Tea
Nettle Tea • Red Raspberry Leaf Tea • Hibiscus Iced Tea
Ginger Tea • Labor Tea • Postpartum Tea • Bedtime Sleepy Milk

¼ cup hot filtered water

I teaspoon tamarind paste
(available in Asian food
stores)

¼ teaspoon chili powder

Pinch of salt

I tablespoon brown sugar

½ ripe mango, peeled,
pitted, and thinly sliced

I apple, peeled, cored, and
thinly sliced

½ ripe-but-firm papaya,
peeled, seeded, and cubed

I cup cubed fresh or canned
(unsweetened) pineapple

Rujak

SERVES 4 TO 6

Women in Bali introduced me to rujak as a cure for nausea when I was expecting my youngest, Hanoman. There were days when I just could not keep food down. Since I knew the baby and I needed to be nourished, I felt terrible. Eating a small serving of rujak seemed to light my digestive fires. The nausea would recede and, after a short while, I would be able to eat protein and grains. In late pregnancy, rujak helped me cope with heartburn.

In a small bowl, mix the water with the tamarind paste until the paste is dissolved. Add the chili powder, salt, and sugar; mix well. In a large bowl, toss the tamarind sauce with the mangos, apple, papaya, and pineapple and serve.

Fruit Salad

SERVES 4 TO 6

This salad is full of vitamins, minerals, and calcium. To choose fruit for the salad, use your imagination and check your yard trees for ripe fruit.

In a small bowl, mix the yogurt, lime juice, and honey. In a large bowl, gently toss the fruit and coconut with the yogurt sauce. Serve and enjoy.

6 cups assorted sliced or diced fruits in season, such as papaya, banana, mango, peaches, pears, apples, raspberries, strawberries, mulberries, kiwi fruit, oranges (peeled with sections broken into pieces), and green or red grapes

Dried, grated coconut

1½ cups plain yogurt

½ teaspoon fresh lime or lemon juice

1 teaspoon raw honey

Banana Raita

SERVES 4

2 to 3 ripe bananas, sliced into bite-size rounds

1½ cups plain yogurt

1 teaspoon ground cardamom

½ teaspoon ground ginger

Serve raita as a side dish with any rice-based meal, or by itself as a snack. The cardamom will help you digest the bananas, and the ginger will help you digest the yogurt, which is an important source of calcium and protein.

In a medium serving bowl, combine the bananas with the yogurt, cardamom, and ginger. Allow to stand for a few minutes so the flavors develop, and then serve.

Pear Salad

SERVES 4

2 to 3 very ripe pears, cored and cubed

1 to 2 cups cottage cheese

1 generous handful of alfalfa sprouts

This variation on the cottage cheese and pear salad is made with fresh pears. Cottage cheese is a perfect food to keep on hand for when you need a quick calcium or protein fix: It's simple, fast, and satisfying.

Arrange the pears on individual salad plates and surround with sprouts. Top with a scoop of cottage cheese for each plate. Serve immediately.

Simple Papaya

SERVES 1 TO 2

Papayas contain papain, an enzyme that supports diges-tion. This delicious fruit is rich in vitamin C and beta-carotene, which helps you obtain the vitamin A you need. The addition of a squeeze of lime or lemon provides the healing power of citrus fruit. This is a good nausea buster in early pregnancy. In late pregnancy, when heartburn sets in, papaya can really help.

Squeeze the lime over the fruit. Serve with a spoon.

I lime wedge

I papaya, halved lengthwise and seeded

Lychee Nut Balls

SERVES 4 TO 6

This is a "just for fun" treat; however, the cream cheese does provide calcium and a good protein pick-me-up.

Stuff the lychees with cream cheese. Serve.

I (20-ounce) can lychees (available in Asian markets), drained

4 ounces cream cheese

4 to 5 ripe frozen bananas (more if they are small)

4 to 5 tablespoons roasted almond butter

2 teaspoons natural almond extract (sold in health-food stores)

Filtered water

Almond–Banana Smoothie

SERVES 4

Almonds are nearly 20 percent protein. They are high in vitamin B, vitamin E, calcium, copper, iron, zinc, potassium, phosphorus, manganese, magnesium, and selenium. According to Chinese medicine, almonds cure hemorrhoids. Ayurvedic healing teaches us that almonds are warming, tonic, and reduce "vata" (wind and space in the body). Bananas provide potassium, iron, magnesium, and selenium. Freeze the bananas the day before you prepare smoothies. This is a perfect way to use your overripe bananas. (But for the first 6 weeks postpartum, avoid overly cold foods. Make the smoothie with 3 to 4 unfrozen bananas and one frozen one.)

Combine the bananas in a blender with the almond butter and almond extract. Add enough water to fill the blender to 2 inches below its brim. Blend until smooth and creamy. Serve immediately.

Alesia's Life-Saving Date Shake

SERVES 2

Alesia, mom of Charan and Shanti, is known for her artistic passion. She feels this nourishing, easy-to-digest drink brings her into balance. Serves one hungry new mother or two regular folks.

In a medium saucepan, slowly bring the milk, ghee, rosewater, date, and raisins to a boil. Let cool; you want it warm, not scalding hot. Add the cardamom, cinnamon, and ginger. Pour the mixture into a blender. Blend until smooth, and enjoy.

2 cups milk

1/4 teaspoon ghee (see page 198)

5 to 6 drops rosewater (available in Asian groceries and health-food stores)

1 Medjool date or 2 small dates

1/4 cup raisins

Pinch of ground cardamom

Pinch of ground cinnamon

Pinch of ground ginger

I cup plain yogurt

2 cups filtered water

I ripe mango, peeled, pitted, and chopped

Pinch of ground cardamom

3 to 4 dates (optional)

Rose petals (unsprayed from your garden), for garnish

Aam or Mango Lassi

SERVES 2

Lassi is taken by itself or sipped after a meal. It is a digestive aid and (as it is so delicious) a mood booster. The dates are an optional extra for those with a sweet tooth! Choose soft ones and remove pits.

Combine the yogurt, water, mango, cardamom, and dates in a blender. Blend until smooth and creamy. Serve garnished with rose petals.

"I have never met anyone who could not drink lassi."

DR. B.D. TRIGUNA

Summertime Smoothie

SERVES 2

Our dear friend Alesia keeps her eyes bright and her heart open with this nutritious warm weather drink. It's creamy but dairy-free.

Combine all the ingredients in a blender and blend until smooth. Serve immediately.

6 to 8 ounces strawberry-flavored soy yogurt

1 banana

1 cup soy milk

¾ cup fresh or frozen berries, such as strawberries, blueberries, mulberries, boysenberries, or raspberries

½ cup apple juice

Engorged Breasts?
Try a Hot Ginger Compress

*M*any breastfeeding mothers occasionally suffer from painfully engorged breasts. Often this is caused by stress and lack of rest. For instant relief, make a ginger root compress.

1. Grate a 2-inch knot of fresh ginger.

2. Place in a medium-sized bowl.

3. Pour approximately 1 cup of boiling water over the ginger.

4. Make a compress by soaking a clean cotton cloth in the ginger water.

5. Apply as warm as you can, without causing discomfort, directly to the affected breast.

Remember, rest will help you recuperate.

¾ cup raw almonds

2 tablespoons sesame seeds

6 ounces soft silken tofu

¼ cup plain yogurt

I banana, frozen and cut
into chunks

I cup frozen strawberries
(frozen raspberries or
mixed berries are also
good)

½ to I cup plain or vanilla
soy milk

Sammy's Silken Tofu Smoothie

SERVES 2

While working for Volunteers in Asia, we met Sam. Soon he and my Balinese daughter, Ketut Rusni (actually daughter of my best friends in Bali) fell in love. Five years later, Ketut and Sam were married and living in Maui, where their first son, Wayan Prajna, was born. I was honored to be on hand for the birth. In the last days of Ketut's pregnancy, Sam would make this smoothie before running off to teach school. Full of protein, calcium, and vitamins, it's so nutritious, it's brilliant!

Soak the almonds and sesame seeds overnight in filtered water to cover. In the morning, drain the nuts and seeds and place them in the blender. Add the tofu, yogurt, banana, berries, and ½ cup soy milk and blend until smooth. You may need to add the remaining ½ cup soy milk to create a "smoothie" consistency. Enjoy the rich, creamy, and flavorful quality of this "meal in a blender."

Avocado-Kiwi Cooler

SERVES 2

Kiwi fruit is high in vitamin C and potassium. Add to that all the benefits of eating avocados and the health benefits of yogurt. (Yogurt aids digestion and provides B vitamins and calcium.)

In a medium bowl, gently mix the avocado, kiwi, and yogurt together. Serve with a sprig of mint.

I ripe avocado, peeled and cubed

2 ripe kiwi fruit, peeled and sliced

I cup plain yogurt

2 mint sprigs (optional)

Sources of Bioflavonoids

Citrus fruits, such as lemons, limes, grapefruits, oranges, and tangerines, are good sources of bioflavonoids. Go ahead and eat the pulp and the white of the rind, where the bioflavonoids are concentrated.

Other good sources of "vitamin P" include apricots, cherries, grapes, black currants, plums, blackberries, papayas, tomatoes, and rose hips. Also, you will find it in green peppers and broccoli.

Caffeine-Free Chai

SERVES 4 TO 6

3 cups milk (cow, goat, soy,
or rice milk)

3 cups filtered water

1 large cinnamon stick,
broken into smaller
pieces

4 to 6 whole cloves

2 pieces star anise

1 (1-inch) piece fresh ginger,
thinly sliced

2 to 4 cardamom pods,
crushed

Vanilla bean (optional)

5 to 6 teaspoons raw honey

Chai tea is a traditional beverage in India, where it is loved because it is a delicious digestive aid. When suffering from the most common pregnancy discomforts—nausea and heartburn—sip this soothing tea, warm or cold.

In a medium saucepan, bring the milk, water, cinnamon, cloves, anise, ginger, cardamom, and vanilla to a slow boil. Let it simmer for 7 to 10 minutes on the lowest heat. You may wish to leave it uncovered, as the aroma is divine. Remove from the heat and allow the chai to cool until it is just the right temperature for drinking. Now add the honey. (Remember, honey should never be boiled.) Strain and serve in heavy mugs or allow to cool and serve over ice.

Lemon Tea

SERVES 1

1 to 1½ cups hot or cold
filtered water

1 tablespoon fresh lemon
juice

1 to 2 tablespoons pure
maple syrup

Enjoy this tea hot or cold. It is a good edema preventative and helps resolve it as well. The combination of lemon and pure maple syrup helps to gently clean the kidneys. Sweeten to taste; don't overdo it.

Just mix it up and enjoy. I prefer it with more water, less lemon and maple syrup.

Nettle Tea

A nutritive herb, the nettle (Urtica dioica) *is high in iron as well as many other minerals, and vitamins C, D, K, and A. It is a specific cure for anemia associated with pregnancy and it helps prevent high blood pressure. It is recommended to minimize varicose veins as it heals the renal and vascular systems of the body. If you suffer from varicose veins (in the legs, vulva, vagina, or rectum [where they are better known as hemorrhoids]), do not massage them. Drink 1 to 2 cups of nettle tea per day. There are no contraindications for the use of nettles in pregnancy or while breastfeeding.*

Combine the nettles and water and allow to steep or infuse for 4 to 6 hours (or overnight) in a covered jar or tea pot (so nutrients don't escape with the steam). Strain and serve warm or at room temperature.

2 ounces dried nettle leaves (available in health-food stores) or 2 generous handfuls of cut-up fresh leaves (handled with care)

8 cups filtered water, boiling

2 ounces dried red raspberry leaves (available in health-food stores) or 2 generous handfuls of cut-up fresh leaves

8 cups filtered water, boiling

2 tablespoons of raw honey

Red Raspberry Leaf Tea

The red raspberry leaf is a tonic for the uterus and, in my opinion, the "queen" of herbs for enhancing pregnancy. Its benefits include increased fertility, prevention of miscarriage, alleviation of morning sickness, reduction of the pain of labor and afterbirth, increased uterine function (which is a component of safe and speedy birthing). It also helps the uterus effectively birth the placenta and aids in the production of breast milk.

Red raspberry leaves are high in iron, so this tea is good for the prevention and treatment of anemia. It contains vitamins A, C, E, and B complex. It is rich in many minerals including calcium, phosphorus, and potassium.

You can make this tea and the Nettle Tea (on the preceding page) in 1-quart quantities, though I prefer to make more, so I will drink plenty. I also like to mix red raspberry and nettles for a nutritive tonic tea. My entire family enjoys it cold in the summer months.

Combine the raspberry leaves and water and allow to steep or infuse for 4 to 6 hours, or overnight, in a covered jar or tea pot (so nutrients don't escape with the steam). Strain and serve warm or at room temperature.

Hibiscus Iced Tea

SERVES 2 TO 4

Hibiscus flowers are known for their healing properties, especially for the kidneys and female reproductive organs. They are a blood purifier and cooling to the body. I often recommend this for women suffering from itching skin during pregnancy. The hibiscus flowers calm the "fire." In addition, the ginger helps alleviate first-trimester nausea. In later pregnancy, hibiscus flowers can relieve heartburn. Hawaiian, Balinese, Ayurvedic, and Chinese medical traditions all recommend hibiscus for pregnancy.

Bring 2 cups of the water to a boil. Pour it over the hibiscus flowers and ginger. Let steep for 5 minutes. Add 2 cups cold water. Stir in the honey. Once the honey has dissolved, add the remaining 6 cups water. Chill and serve with a sprig of fresh garden mint.

10 cups filtered water

1 ounce dried hibiscus flowers

1 (1-inch piece) fresh ginger, peeled and thinly sliced

2 tablespoons raw honey or more to taste

Sprig fresh mint

I (2-inch) piece fresh ginger, peeled and mashed with a pestle or a stone

4 cups filtered water, boiling

2 to 4 tablespoons raw honey

Squeeze of fresh lime, lemon, or tangerine (optional for additional vitamin C)

Ginger Tea

SERVES 2 TO 4

Ginger is a wonderful aid to digestion—just what you need to sip to alleviate third-trimester heartburn. It also helps relieve first-trimester nausea. In Chinese medicine and Ayurvedic medicine, ginger root is a recommended treatment for colds, flu, indigestion, vomiting, belching, abdominal pain, laryngitis, arthritis, hemorrhoids, headaches, and heart disease. In India it is considered the most sattvic or life- and light-supporting of spices. According to Ayurvedic principles, during pregnancy the wind in our bodies is reversed; this condition supports the growing fetus, but for many women causes pregnancy discomforts. Fresh ginger is nature's best antidote for discomforts due to wind.

Place ginger in a teapot or a quart jar, and pour in the boiling water. Allow to cool. When the tea is lukewarm, stir in the honey (cooking honey destroys its precious nutrients). Add citrus if desired, and serve warm or cold.

Labor Tea

This tea may be sweetened with honey if desired; it really does take the edge off labor pains (according to women in labor) without reducing the effectiveness of the contractions. This tea will also ease the pain of menstrual cramps.

Boil the basil in the water for 2 minutes. Turn off the heat and allow the tea to steep for 20 minutes. Serve warm.

1 handful (about $1/2$ cup packed) fresh basil leaves

2 cups filtered water

Postpartum Tea

SERVES 1

This soothing tea should be made ahead, as it must be served cooled to be effective in reducing postpartum bleeding. This tea is also traditionally used by Mayan healers to alleviate adult diarrhea.

Pour the water over the roses and leaves and allow to steep for 15 minutes. Serve cool.

1 cup filtered water, boiling

3 red roses (fresh organically grown)

9 rose leaves (nine is an important healing number in Mayan tradition)

Labor Tea and Postpartum Tea

These simple, effective recipes come to me via Kathy Warner, who studied under Rosita Arvigo, D. N., a Mayan healer who practices in Belize. I highly recommend Rosita's book (coauthored with Michael Balick, Ph.D.) *Rainforest Remedies*.

2 cups milk

Garam masala, storebought
or homemade (see page
199) (optional)

½ teaspoon ghee (see page
198)

1 teaspoon raw honey

Bedtime Sleepy Milk

SERVES 2

*Ghee (clarified butter), honey, and milk are considered
foods of the gods in India. This combination soothes the
body and promotes a deep, restful sleep. Milk contains the
amino acid tryptophan, which helps alleviate insomnia.
Mother's milk is sweeter and more unctuous (oily) than
cow's milk. Adding ghee and honey to cow's milk makes it
more soothing, just like mother's milk.*

In a saucepan over medium heat, bring the milk to a boil.
If you are adding garam masala to the milk, do so as it
comes to a gentle boil. Remove the milk from the heat and
add the ghee. Allow the mixture to cool further and then
add the honey. Sweet dreams.

SALADS, VEGETABLES, AND SIDES

Vegetables are a rich source of vitamins and minerals for the expectant or breastfeeding woman. Just look at them: their colors tell you how important they are in your daily diet. You will feel so good if you eat plenty of vegetables—gifts from the Mother Earth.

DRESSING

6 tablespoons filtered water

2 tablespoons extra virgin olive oil

2 tablespoons grated Parmesan cheese

1 tablespoon Dijon mustard

1 tablespoon ginger or orange marmalade

1 tablespoon fresh lemon juice

SALAD

1 head romaine lettuce, cut into bite-sized pieces

1 large tomato, cubed

8 ounces assorted sprouts (alfalfa, radish, mung, sunflower, etc.)

4 to 6 ounces feta cheese, cubed or crumbled

1/2 cup pitted kalamata olives

Wednesday Night Salad

SERVES 4 TO 6

This salad comes together very quickly, especially if one person is making the dressing while another is chopping the lettuce. Feta cheese is a good source of protein, and the touch of lemon increases the overall nutritional value. This is a perfect salad to serve with fish and a grain.

Whisk the dressing ingredients together in a deep bowl, or shake together in a jar. Toss the lettuce, tomato, sprouts, feta cheese, and olives together in a large salad bowl. Pour the dressing over all, toss, and serve.

Nephew's Salad

SERVES 4 TO 6

This recipe comes from my nephew Carl. It's as unusual and delightful as the angel wings tattooed on his back. It's also rich in vitamin C, with all the nutrition of nuts as an additional feature.

Toss the lettuce and orange pieces with the nuts. Mix together the oil and lemon juice, and drizzle it over lettuce mixture. Add salt to taste, toss, and serve.

12 to 15 large leaves of leafy green or red lettuce (enough to fill a large salad bowl, cut or torn into pieces just a wee bit larger than bite-sized

2 oranges, peeled, sectioned, seeded, and cut into bite-sized pieces

½ cup walnuts or sunflower seeds

2 tablespoons extra virgin olive oil

2 tablespoons fresh lemon juice

Sea salt

A Few Words about Sprouts

*S*prouted seeds, grains, and beans can be found in most grocery stores today. This is a blessing. When a seed is sprouted, the stored life-force is born, and the protein content increases by 15 to 30 percent.

Sprouting increases the niacin, riboflavin, and beta-carotene (precursor to vitamin A) content of the food. Vitamins C, E, K, calcium, phosphorus, and iron content all go up. When the sprouts begin to get green, the chlorophyll content increases and they become more nutritious. Alfalfa sprouts are easy to find. Try also aduki, buckwheat, clover, fenugreek, garbanzo, green pea, lentil, lima bean, mung, radish, soybean, sunflower, and wheat sprouts.

Whether you eat sprouts on your sandwich, mix them into salad, or just use them as a garnish, this living food will greatly benefit your health and vitality.

SALAD

1 large bunch spinach,
   washed, stemmed, and
   torn into bite-sized pieces

1 (8-ounce) can Mandarin
   orange slices, drained, or
   2 tangerines, peeled,
   seeded, and sectioned

$1/3$ to $1/2$ pound Monterey
   Jack or provolone cheese,
   cubed, or $1/2$ pound firm
   tofu, cubed

$1/2$ cup slivered almonds

DRESSING

$1/2$ cup extra virgin olive oil

$1/4$ cup toasted sesame oil

Juice of $1/2$ lemon

1 ($1/2$-inch) piece fresh
   ginger, grated

2 tablespoons apple cider
   vinegar

1 teaspoon raw honey

2 tablespoons tamari or soy
   sauce

Freshly ground black pepper

Asian Spinach Salad

SERVES 2 TO 4

During pregnancy your calcium needs rise from approximately 1,000 to 1,300 milligrams per day. Breastfeeding women's bodies require around 1,500 milligrams of calcium daily, plus additional amounts of most other nutrients. This salad is calcium-rich due to the inclusion of cheese or tofu. Please shop for an organic cheese or tofu; your body deserves the best.

In a large bowl, toss all of the salad ingredients together. To make the dressing, combine the oils, lemon juice, ginger, vinegar, honey and tamari in a lidded jar and shake until well blended. Pour the dressing over salad and toss some more. Serve with freshly ground pepper to taste.

Mango Cashew Salad

SERVES 6

This salad has a distinctly Asian flavor. I haven't yet met a soul who did not love it. You might toast the cashews ahead of time, or sprinkle them on warm from the skillet. Cashews are a source of magnesium, potassium, iron, zinc, and some calcium, vitamin A, and B vitamins.

Toss the lettuce and mango together in a large wooden salad bowl.

To make the cashew topping, heat a cast-iron skillet over medium heat. Add the cashews, and toast, stirring often, until the cashews begin to brown, about 3 minutes. Add the sugar and salt, and continue to roast while stirring constantly. When the sugar caramelizes and sticks to the nuts, the topping is ready.

To make the dressing, grate the ginger into a small bowl. Add the oils, tamari, and vinegar and whisk with a fork. Pour the dressing over salad, sprinkle the cashew topping on top, and toss. Serve and get ready for compliments.

I head romaine lettuce (or any organic salad mix of your choice) torn into bite-size pieces

I ripe mango, peeled, pitted, and cubed

CASHEW TOPPING

I cup raw cashew halves or pieces

I tablespoon raw sugar or Sucanat

1/8 teaspoon sea salt

DRESSING

I (1 1/2-inch) piece fresh ginger, peeled

1/4 cup almond or extra virgin olive oil

I tablespoon toasted sesame oil

I tablespoon plus I teaspoon tamari or soy sauce

1/4 cup rice or apple cider vinegar

3 large apples

3 large carrots

½ cup raisins

DRESSING

¼ cup extra virgin olive oil

¼ teaspoon sea salt

½ teaspoon raw honey

Juice of ½ lemon

1 cup alfalfa sprouts, for garnish

Christina's Apple Salad

SERVES 4 TO 6

What a joy it is to visit Christina's house. Her three children, ages three to eight, are being home-schooled. Devan can be heard playing the piano. His sister, Erika, is busy telling a story to her little brother, Rowan, at the flannel board. As lunchtime approaches, Christina begins in the kitchen and the children wander in to help out. It is a simple and joyful way to learn sound nutrition.

Using a stainless-steel grater, grate the apples and carrots into a medium bowl and toss with the raisins. In a small bowl, whisk together the oil, salt, honey, and lemon juice to make a sauce. Add the sauce to the carrot mixture and toss with two forks. Garnish with the sprouts. Serve as a side dish with a meal or by itself as a snack.

Beet Salad

SERVES 2

This calcium-rich salad-snack is also a liver cleanser. The omega-3 fatty acids in flaxseed oil are good for fetal brain development, so eat this often.

Peel and grate the beet. Add flaxseed oil, lemon juice, tamari, and sesame seeds, and toss. Divide between two plates. Garnish with mint and share with your partner.

I large beet

I tablespoon flaxseed oil

½ teaspoon fresh lemon or lime juice

½ teaspoon tamari or soy sauce

I teaspoon toasted sesame seeds or sesame gomashio (see page 198)

2 sprigs mint, for garnish

Getting into the Garden...

*F*ew pleasures are as satisfying as gardening. I figure my little vegetable, herb, and flower patch has provided me with tens of thousands of dollars worth of therapy. When I feel out-of-sorts or blue, I head for the garden and get my hands into the soil. Mother Earth is always there for me. The food and bounty my family reaps from our garden nourishes our souls and our bodies. My granddaughter loves to work in the garden. When my husband Wil and I have worries, we get out in the garden. When I feel one of the children needs individual attention, we grab a couple of spades and get digging. What an education the garden has been, as well as grounding, beautiful, and bountiful.

6 to 8 small beets, peeled
and cut into bite-size
pieces

1 tablespoon butter or ghee
(see page 198)

1 (½-inch) piece fresh
ginger, peeled and diced

2 cloves garlic, crushed, or
pinch of hing (see Note)

1 cup fresh orange juice

2 teaspoons raw sugar or
Sucanat

2 teaspoons arrowroot
powder or cornstarch

1 generous handful of fresh
mint, minced, or 2
teaspoons dried mint

Marjan's Favorite Beets

SERVES 4 TO 6

Marjan, a native of the Netherlands, prepared this beet dish while pregnant and breastfeeding her daughter. Beets are calcium-rich and, with the addition of savory spices, are deliciously easy to digest. Try serving them with Christine's Dijon Green Quiche (page 142).

Steam the beets until they are tender, about 10 to 12 minutes, and set them aside.

In a medium saucepan over low heat, melt the butter. Add the ginger and garlic, if using and sauté for about 1 minute.

Stir together the orange juice, sugar, and arrowroot powder, until dissolved. Whisk the orange juice mixture into the ginger-butter and continue to simmer and whisk until thickened, about 3 to 5 minutes.

Pour the sauce over the beets and toss with the mint. Serve hot or cold.

Note: Hing is an herb that is also known as asafetida; it is available wherever Asian or Indian foods are sold. You should avoid garlic and hing during the first six weeks postpartum.

Warm Shiitake Mushroom Salad

SERVES 2 TO 4

This recipe comes to us from the Ruins Café, in Baguio City, Philippines, my mother's hometown. I've made it for friends in Iowa, Bali, and Paris, and they all were amazed at how delicious and satisfying it is. I serve it as a main dish, with a side of tofu for added protein. This is a great way to get all eight essential amino acids into one dish.

If you are using dried shiitakes, rehydrate by soaking in cold water for 2 hours. Or pour boiling water over and soak for 15 to 20 minutes. Remove from the soaking liquid and pat dry.

In a wok or cast-iron skillet, warm the sesame oil over medium heat and place the mushrooms, tops facing down, in the pan. In a small bowl, mix together the ginger, sesame seeds, lime juice, and tamari. Pour some of this sauce into each mushroom, and add the water to the bottom of the pan. Cover and allow to simmer over low heat for 15 minutes, until the mushrooms are tender and well cooked. Make sure the pan does not dry out and burn the mushrooms. If the pan begins to dry out, add more water.

Arrange the watercress on individual plates. Place a few mushrooms on top of each plate of greens, and garnish with the snow peas and avocado. Pour the remaining sauce over the mushrooms. Serve warm.

8 to 10 fresh or dried shiitake mushrooms, stemmed

3 tablespoons toasted sesame oil

1 (1-inch) piece fresh ginger, peeled and grated

1 tablespoon sesame seeds

2 tablespoons fresh lime or lemon juice

3 tablespoons tamari or soy sauce

1/4 cup filtered water

1 large bunch watercress (about 1 pound), torn into bite-size pieces (or substitute red or green leaf lettuce)

1/2 cup snow peas, strings removed (optional)

1 avocado, peeled, pitted, and sliced (optional)

2 cups plain yogurt

¼ cup whipping cream

I cucumber, peeled, seeded, and diced or grated

Kernels cut from I ear sweet corn

2 teaspoons ground coriander

I teaspoon ground cumin

¼ teaspoon dill seed—fresh if available, or dried

½ teaspoon toasted fennel seed

½ teaspoon sea salt

¼ teaspoon curry powder

¼ cup chopped fresh cilantro

2 tablespoons chopped fresh mint

Pinch of raw sugar or Sucanat

Raita à la Megan

SERVES 4 TO 6

Raita is a wonderful digestive aid, plus it adds protein and calcium to any meal. This version of raita was invented by Megan (mother of Corwin). It is so wonderful and much more exotic than the typical version. Serve it with lentils or curry dishes.

Mix all the ingredients in a medium bowl. Serve at once.

Getting Children to Eat Salad

I discovered that many flowers are edible and delicious, too. Adding edible flowers to salads really makes them more appealing to my children. Maybe it will work for you, too. When I plant my spring garden I include edible flowers in the planning. Did you know you can eat pansies? How about daylilies? Some flowers taste a bit peppery but that has never discouraged my children, who eat flowers with delight. My granddaughter calls salad that includes flowers "Fairy Salad." Finely diced mint leaves, tossed right in the salad with the greens makes "Fairy Salad" particularly refreshing.

White Cabbage Salad

SERVES 4 TO 6

I find that whenever I'm feeling a little off-balance, I crave vinegar. This dish is a good pick-me-up.

Combine the water, vinegar, caraway, salt, and pepper in a nonreactive saucepan. Bring to a boil, lower the heat, and allow to simmer for about 3 minutes. Place the cabbage in a large bowl. Pour the vinegar mixture, hot, over the cabbage. Now, using a wooden spoon, press hard on the cabbage to compact it in the bowl. Let it sit and marinate for at least 1 hour.

Arrange turkey bacon slices to lie flat in a cast-iron skillet. On medium heat cook until crisp, turn and crisp second side. Set aside, cool, and crumble.

Mix the crumbled bacon, oil, and wine, in a cup or small bowl. Toss this mixture through the marinated cabbage. *Guten Appetit!*

I cup filtered water

¼ cup balsamic or apple cider vinegar

½ teaspoon ground caraway or cumin

I teaspoon sea salt

½ teaspoon freshly ground black pepper

I pound white or green cabbage, finely sliced (approximately 3 to 4 cups)

4 slices turkey bacon

½ cup extra virgin olive oil

2 tablespoons red wine (optional)

1 teaspoon cumin seeds

2 cucumbers, peeled and
  diced

1½ cups plain yogurt

Sea salt

Cucumber Raita

SERVES 4

This recipe helps balance new mothers because cucumber, which is sweet and astringent, decreases the "vata" or wind in the body. The yogurt is a good source of protein. It's also good for digestion and alleviates diarrhea and painful urination.

Roast the cumin seeds in a dry cast-iron skillet or frying pan for approximately 2 minutes on medium heat. When aromatic and brown, place the seeds on a cutting board and crush with a rolling pin. Mix the cumin, cucumbers, and yogurt in a medium-sized serving bowl. Add salt to taste. Allow to sit for half an hour before serving, to allow the flavors to marry.

Lebanese Potato Salad

SERVES 6 TO 8

Rebecca, mother of Inti, is truly an international daughter. Her mother's family is from the Netherlands. Her father's family hails from Lebanon. She grew up in Iowa. I can always depend upon Rebecca to come up with something delicious to eat. If she can't remember the recipe, she picks up the phone and gets the details from her family. This Lebanese version of potato salad is wonderful. To really enjoy the flavors make it the day before you plan to serve it. Rebecca uses organic potatoes and does not peel them, to get the full nutritional benefit.

Put potatoes in a large lidded pot with enough water to cover them; boil for 15 to 20 minutes or more until tender but not falling apart. Drain, set aside to cool. When potatoes are at room temperature combine the potatoes, parsley, garlic, and lemon juice in a large bowl. Toss the ingredients together until well blended. Drizzle with olive oil and season with salt and pepper to taste. Cover and refrigerate. Serve the next day with the chutney on the side.

5 pounds white potatoes, boiled and cubed

1 bunch Italian parsley, finely chopped

6 to 8 cloves garlic, minced

Juice of 4 lemons

¾ cup extra virgin olive oil

Sea salt

Freshly ground black pepper

Middle Eastern Mint Chutney (page 202)

6 medium to large white- or
   orange-fleshed sweet
   potatoes

½ to ¾ cup mayonnaise

¼ cup tamari or soy sauce

1 medium yellow onion,
   finely diced

3 to 4 celery stalks, diced

1 (6-inch) piece pickled
   daikon radish, quartered
   lengthwise and diced

Freshly ground black pepper

2 sheets roasted nori
   seaweed, for garnish

Asian Potato Salad

SERVES 4 TO 6

As a child I loved my father's German potato salad recipe. That love led me to experiment with an Asian version. Aboriginal Australians consider sweet potatoes and yams "medicine" for pregnant and postpartum women. Sweet potatoes are high in beta-carotene, with vitamin C and A, B vitamins, iron, and potassium, and yams include folic acid, potassium, and magnesium, plus vitamins.

You might want to try this recipe with Okinawan sweet potatoes, which have white skins and violet flesh—so lovely! Try finding them, as well as pickled daikon, at Asian markets and natural food stores or local organic farms. My family loves this salad as a side dish at spring picnics or summer barbecues.

Boil the sweet potatoes in water to cover until well done but not mushy, 7 to 10 minutes. Drain and allow the sweet potatoes to cool. Once they've cooled, cut into bite-size pieces. In a large salad bowl, combine the mayonnaise and tamari. Combine the onion, celery, and daikon together, and fold into mayo-tamari mixture until well blended. Add the sweet potatoes and stir until potatoes are covered with dressing. Season with black pepper to taste and refrigerate until chilled. Just before serving crumble the nori seaweed on top of the salad.

Streets of Taiwan Tomato Salad

SERVES 2 TO 4

Nina Tichy, a dear friend from Taiwan, taught me to make this salad, which she enjoyed as a child and is a common street food in Taiwan. I have also found it at the food courts in Singapore. I often tell pregnant women who are suffering from indigestion and heartburn to eat many small meals, rather that three large meals per day. When you use the tofu in this dish, it becomes one of those perfect small meals.

In a medium bowl, toss the tomatoes with the tamari, sesame oil, and ginger. Add the tofu. Serve as a summertime side dish.

2 large ripe tomatoes, sliced into wedges

2 tablespoons tamari or soy sauce

I tablespoon toasted sesame oil

I (I-inch) piece fresh ginger, peeled and grated

1/2 pound firm tofu, cubed (optional)

½ pound fresh mozzarella cheese, cubed

8 to 12 leaves fresh basil, sliced into fine strips

1 teaspoon dried oregano

1 clove garlic, minced

4 medium ripe tomatoes, diced

2 to 4 tablespoons extra virgin olive oil

Sea salt

Caprese

SERVES 4

This protein-rich salad dish is a good quick fix when you need protein fast. Special thanks to Gina Sitz, who e-mailed it to me from Bali.

Combine the cheese, basil, oregano, garlic, tomatoes, and oil in a serving bowl and season to taste with salt. Toss gently. Serve immediately.

Greek Salad

SERVES 6 OR MORE

This is a nutritious salad that can be served by itself. You can make a lot, serve some immediately, and store the rest in the refrigerator so you can snack on it later. Whole-grain pasta is a good source of fuel for new mothers, because it's a complex carbohydrate and contains more nutrients than white pasta.

Cook pasta in approximately 7 pints of boiling water with 2 tablespoons salt, for 8 to 12 minutes, depending upon pasta (follow package directions), stirring often. Try a piece of pasta every so often to see if it is cooked. When desired doneness is achieved, drain quickly. Allow to cool.

Combine all the salad ingredients in a large bowl and toss together.

Combine all the dressing ingredients in a small jar and shake well. Toss with the salad and serve.

SALAD

1 pound rainbow or whole-wheat pasta curls or shells

2 tablespoons sea salt

1 pound feta cheese, cut into bite-sized cubes

1 cup skinless chicken, cooked and cubed, (optional)

1 large ripe tomato, diced

1 generous handful of fresh basil leaves, minced

1 cucumber, peeled and sliced

1 zucchini, sliced

4 ounces assorted sprouts (approximately 1½ cups)

½ cup pitted kalamata olives

¼ cup pitted green olives (pimento-stuffed olives are fine)

¼ to ½ cup grated Parmesan cheese

DRESSING

⅓ cup extra virgin olive oil

2 tablespoons fresh lemon juice or apple cider vinegar

1 clove garlic, grated or minced

½ teaspoon fruit jam or marmalade

Pinch of freshly ground black pepper

Pinch of sea salt

Rainbow Salad

SERVES 6 TO 8

Jacqueline, Camille, Sofia, and Olivia are blessed to be the children of Dean and Christine Goodale. These children eat hardy organic foods, lovingly made by their parents, and the entire family has a healthy glow. Rainbow Salad is one brilliant way to get your children to eat veggies. The tangy dressing makes this salad unique and flavorful. The colors will astound your eyes and enliven your table or picnic.

In a large salad bowl, toss together the cilantro, beet, carrots, corn, rice, eggs, pumpkin seeds, and raisins. In a small lidded jar, combine the dressing ingredients and shake well. Pour the dressing over the salad, toss, and garnish with alfalfa sprouts. Serve immediately.

SALAD

½ bunch cilantro or parsley, chopped (stems may be included if chopped very finely)

I large beet, peeled and grated

2 medium carrots, grated

Kernels cut from 2 ears corn

I cup cooked brown rice

2 to 3 hard-boiled eggs, peeled and cubed

¼ cup roasted pumpkin seeds

¼ cup raisins

Alfalfa sprouts, for garnish

DRESSING

2 tablespoons apple cider or balsamic vinegar

¼ cup extra virgin olive oil

½ teaspoon raw sugar or Sucanat

I small clove garlic, finely minced

I tablespoon tamari or soy sauce

I to 2 tablespoons nutritional yeast

Pop-Pop Hemmerle's Mashed Roots

SERVES 6 TO 8

My father-in-love is known for his cooking. Many a Sunday afternoon he prepares a "home-cooked" meal for the elder men who gather at the VFW Hall in Barrington, New Jersey. This version of mashed potatoes is protein-rich and more nutritious than traditional mashed potatoes. My children just love it. Each time I gave birth, the first food I wanted to eat afterward was a huge bowl of mashed root vegetables, smothered in butter and served in my favorite deep blue bowl. This is comfort food at its best.

Since most of the protein in potatoes is just underneath the skin, I don't remove the peel. Put the potatoes and carrots in a big pot; add enough water to just cover them. Boil until tender, about 15 minutes. Drain nearly all the water off (I often save this water for soup). Drop the butter in pieces into drained hot potatoes and carrots. Begin to mash. In a separate bowl beat the eggs with the milk. Add to the potatoes and continue to mash until fluffy. Add salt and pepper to taste. The heat of the potatoes will cook the egg, and your family will not even notice it. Garnish with sprouts for additional nutrients.

10 or 12 large russet potatoes, peeled (optional) and cubed

3 to 4 large carrots, cut into 1/2-inch rounds

1/2 cup (1 stick) butter

2 large eggs

1 1/2 cups whole milk

Sea salt and freshly ground black pepper

Sprouts, to garnish

I tablespoon extra virgin
   olive oil

3 medium or 4 small beets,
   peeled, halved, and thinly
   sliced

I large bunch kale or your
   favorite green, stemmed,
   washed, and cut into
   pieces slightly bigger
   than bite size
   (approximately 4 cups,
   packed)

I tablespoon tamari or soy
   sauce

Juice of ½ small lemon

¾ cup grated sharp cheddar
   cheese

Can't Beet It

SERVES 4

Root vegetables grow right in Mother Earth, where she packs them with vitamins and minerals. Just look at them: You can see they are nutritious by their vivid colors. This iron-rich side dish combines hearty beets with cheese and leafy green vegetables for added calcium and minerals. If your beets are fresh from the garden and still have their tops, don't discard them. Cut the tops up and cook them with the kale.

Fill a wok or large frying pan with a tight-fitting lid with ½ to 1 inch of filtered water. Add the oil and beets and cover. Simmer the beets over medium heat until tender, approximately 10 minutes. Periodically check the beets to be sure the water has not cooked off; add water as needed to avoid burning. Add the kale, cover, and let the greens steam for 2 to 3 minutes until just done. To avoid over-cooking, remove from heat while the kale is still bright green. Toss with tamari, lemon juice, and grated cheese. Serve hot.

Ibu Ana's Roasted Vegetables

SERVES 6 TO 8

What could be more nourishing or healthy than roasted vegetables? Ibu Ana provides us with this wonderful and simple recipe. It keeps her drumming and bicycling at 73! Our children love these vegetables with organic sour cream. This makes a great summertime food to eat out on the picnic table.

Preheat the oven to 350°F. Combine the sweet potatoes, beets, potatoes, carrots and onions, in a large bowl. Coat with oil, spread out on baking sheets, and sprinkle with salt and herbs. Roast, turning the vegetables with a spatula every 15 minutes. When the potatoes are nearly tender, about 45 minutes to 1 hour, add the mushrooms and garlic cloves, return the baking sheets to the oven, and roast again until all are tender, approximately 20 minutes. Serve warm.

4 sweet potatoes, cut into 1-inch cubes

2 large beets, peeled and cut into 1-inch cubes

4 russet potatoes, cut into 1-inch cubes (omit these in the first 6 weeks postpartum)

12 to 15 baby carrots

2 large red onions, quartered (optional)

Extra virgin olive oil

Sea salt

Herbs, dried and ground: oregano, basil, rosemary, or any herbs you love, such as tarragon, marjoram, etc.

12 or more whole button mushrooms

2 garlic heads, broken into cloves, unpeeled (optional)

1 carrot

¼ pound green beans, trimmed

¼ pound snow peas, strings removed

1 broccoli stalk (peel) plus one broccoli head

1 celery stalk

1 large sweet potato, peeled and cubed

1 large potato, peeled and cubed

¼ pound mung bean sprouts

½ pound firm tofu, cubed

SAUCE

½ cup natural peanut butter

¼ cup filtered water

1 tablespoon tamari or soy sauce

¼ teaspoon ground chili powder

½ teaspoon dark brown sugar

1 (½-inch) piece fresh ginger, peeled and grated

Gado-Gado

SERVES 4 TO 6

This nutritious recipe is a traditional Indonesian medley of flavors. Peanuts provide protein, tofu is calcium-rich, and sweet potatoes are nourishing for the female reproductive system. If you prefer, try substituting roasted cashew or almond butter for peanut butter.

Cut the carrot, green beans, snow peas, broccoli, and celery into bite-size pieces. Combine the sweet potato, potato, broccoli stalk, and carrot in a steamer, and steam for 5 minutes until tender, but not soft. Add the green beans, snow peas, broccoli head, and celery and steam for an additional 3 minutes. Add the bean sprouts and tofu, if desired and steam 1 more minute. Remove from the heat and arrange on a platter.

To make the sauce, combine the peanut butter, water, tamari, chili powder, brown sugar, and ginger in a small bowl. Use a fork to stir until smooth. Add more water if necessary, so the sauce will pour. To serve, pour the peanut sauce over the entire lovely mess of vegetables.

As a Child in the Religion of Gratitude

After the frost
has stolen vine and green
tomatoes and hyssop flowers from
    the garden,

After I have piled
dead leaves on,
put away rakes and hung the rusty spade
on two nails in the shed,
—the one you had planned to scrape
    and paint—

After breath comes out white
and curls whistling around blue ears
like a ghost on All Soul's Day,
a familiar spirit
not particularly loved, but not feared,

Still, the bookkeeper mind
cannot understand the color of
    forgiveness.

I go late, intending to make
a new moon soup.
Onion and split peas already in the
    crockery pot.
I pray for a few carrots
in the dark.
In my long coat
I push back dry leaves and move aside
    the crackle.
Removing gloves I find the cold soil
    loose.
Fingers swim and play a minute
before finding four fat carrots.
Is this the color of patience?

So through the wicked season, the
    deep water
keeps muddy frogs alive.
So perhaps the ladybugs, hiding in cracks
on the south sides of old buildings, have
    a little hope.
And so, I've learned tonight, that after
    the frost
there may yet be roots to eat.

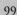

99

I large red cabbage, cored
and diced

4 large apples, peeled, cored,
and diced

2 large red onions, diced

¼ cup extra virgin olive oil

¼ cup filtered water

¼ cup apple cider vinegar

I tablespoon raw sugar or
Sucanat

I teaspoon sea salt

4 to 6 bay leaves

8 to 12 whole cloves

Hannelore's German Winter Cabbage

SERVES 10 TO 15

This dish also comes to us by way of our dear "Ibu Ana." She prepared it for our Christmas dinner one snowy winter, and it was a big hit with the children and the adults. To be really delicious, it must be prepared one day in advance. Warm it up when you are ready to serve it. This warming dish is alive with vitamins and minerals.

In a large stainless steel pot, toss together the cabbage, apples, and onions. Sprinkle oil over all. Toss well. Set aside for 1 hour or more. Add the water, vinegar, sugar, salt, bay leaves, and cloves. Simmer over low heat until the cabbage is tender, but not mushy. Serve warm or at room temperature.

Savory Sweet Red Cabbage

SERVES 4 TO 6

This recipe comes from the expatriate moms of Bali, Indonesia. It's a savory side dish that can be served both warm and cold. The combination of sweet and savory flavors can help alleviate pregnancy-related nausea.

In a large bowl, mix the cabbage and apple with the salt, pepper, caraway, bay leaf, lemon juice, and orange juice. Set aside to marinate.

In a large wok or large pot with a lid, heat the oil to medium-low with the sugar until the sugar dissolves (about 1 to 2 minutes). Add the onion and cook until golden (about 3 minutes). Add the marinated cabbage mixture. Combine gently but thoroughly. Cover and allow the cabbage to steam for 4 to 6 minutes. Meanwhile, whisk the wine, vinegar, and flour in a small bowl. When the cabbage is just about done, add the wine sauce. Combine gently, cover, and cook a few more minutes until sauce becomes translucent. Serve immediately.

I small red cabbage, sliced thinly

I large apple, peeled and sliced

I teaspoon sea salt

$\frac{1}{2}$ teaspoon freshly ground black pepper

I$\frac{1}{2}$ teaspoons ground caraway seeds

I bay leaf

Juice from $\frac{1}{2}$ lemon

Juice from I large orange

2 to 3 tablespoons extra virgin olive oil

I tablespoon raw sugar or Sucanat

I medium white or yellow onion, finely diced

$\frac{1}{2}$ cup red wine

I tablespoon balsamic or apple cider vinegar

I tablespoon flour (whole-wheat, white pastry, spelt)

I pound carrots, diced

Filtered water, enough to cover carrots

2 tablespoons extra virgin olive oil

Raw sesame seed for toasting (see note), or toasted sesame seeds

Baked Sesame Carrots

SERVES 4

This dish is simple, easy to make, and rich in calcium.

Preheat the oven to 350°F. In a medium saucepan, boil the carrots until lightly cooked, about 3 to 4 minutes. Remove from the heat and drain. Toss the carrots with the oil and sesame seeds. Transfer to a covered baking dish and bake for 15 minutes. Serve hot.

Note: To toast the sesame seeds heat a cast-iron skillet until hot. Reduce the flame to low, place the seeds in a skillet. Toss them continuously in the skillet until they begin to pop and turn a light golden color (about 1 minute). Transfer the seeds to a plate and spread them out in a single layer to cool.

Quick Cauliflower

SERVES 4 TO 6

This is a quick side dish. We like it served over a whole grain, such as brown rice or quinoa, with a green salad. If it is true that "you are what you eat," we could all use some cauliflower, which is a head made of hundreds of compact flowers. It is rich in potassium, folic acid, and vitamin C, and contains protein. This "flower" is also a cancer preventive.

In a large cast-iron skillet with a tight-fitting lid, heat the oil over medium heat (don't allow it to smoke). Add the cauliflower and tofu, and top with the turmeric. Salt to taste. Stir-fry for 1 to 2 minutes. Add the water, cover, and allow the steam to finish cooking the dish. It is done when the cauliflower is tender, not mushy. Serve hot.

2 tablespoons toasted sesame or extra virgin olive oil

I head cauliflower, core removed, cut into bite-size pieces

½ pound firm tofu, cut into bite-size pieces

I teaspoon ground turmeric

Sea salt

¼ cup filtered water

1 bunch kale (or your choice of leafy greens) stemmed and chopped into bite-size pieces

1 teaspoon apple cider vinegar

Sea salt

Marina's Leafy Greens

SERVES 4

Leafy greens are full of iron, which every woman needs, especially when she's expecting a baby. Midwives tend to be "spies," always noticing how women are doing nutritionally. Yes, we've been known to peek into your refrigerators to see whether it's harboring vegetables or candy bars. I noticed my friend Marina would go right for the leafy greens when she was nursing her daughter Aluna. Her simple preparation is just about perfect.

Simply steam the kale or greens, making sure not to overcook them. Sprinkle with the vinegar and season to taste with salt. Serve immediately.

Savory Rainbow Chard

SERVES 4

This dish is full of iron, calcium and vitamin C. It's simply nutritious and delicious.

In a large cast-iron skillet with a lid or in a wok, heat the oil over medium-low heat. Add the chard stems to the pan, then place the leaves on top. Add the water, cover, and allow to steam for about 4 minutes, until the leaves are bright green and the stems retain their rainbow colors. Remove the pan from the heat, squeeze the lemon juice over the chard, and sprinkle with salt. Mix well and serve, garnishing with the toasted pine nuts.

Note: To toast the pine nuts, place them in a skillet over medium-low heat. Toss them continuously in the skillet until they begin to turn a light golden color, about 1 to 3 minutes. Transfer to a plate and spread them out in a single layer to cool.

2 tablespoons extra virgin olive oil

1 bunch (approximately ¾ pound) rainbow chard, stems and leaves chopped separately into bite-sized pieces

¼ cup filtered water

1 tablespoon fresh lemon juice

Pinch of sea salt

2 tablespoons toasted pine nuts, for garnish (see Note)

1 bunch spinach (regular variety or New Zealand) stemmed and coarsely chopped

½ bunch cilantro, chopped (stems may be used if chopped very finely)

¼ teaspoon cumin seeds

¼ teaspoon coriander seeds

1 tablespoon extra virgin olive oil

Sea salt

1 (4-ounce) package cream cheese, at room temperature

Creamy Spinach

SERVES 4

This recipe was invented by Megan Robinson, a Fairfield, Iowa, mom who takes cooking into the realm of art. It's easy and delicious, and it makes a beautiful side dish.

Wash the spinach and set aside with the cilantro. Crush the cumin and coriander seeds with a mortar and pestle or grind with an herb grinder.

In a wok or large lidded cast-iron skillet, heat the oil over medium heat and add the crushed seeds. Cook for 3 to 5 minutes, until the seeds are light brown. Do not allow the oil to smoke. Carefully, so as not to splatter hot oil, add the spinach and cilantro, cover, and allow to cook over medium heat for 2 minutes. Check the spinach to make sure that it's not too dry. If spinach appears dry, add just a bit of water. Season to taste with salt. Place dots of cream cheese on top of the spinach, cover, and turn off the heat. Allow the dish to sit covered for 5 minutes. The cream cheese will melt, and the spinach will finish steaming. Serve immediately.

Potatoes Sophia

SERVES 4

Sophia and I became dear friends in Bali. I was expecting Hanoman; she was pregnant with Xenia. Over the years we've shared many tears and much laughter. Sophia has illustrated my poetry books, and her art and heart have graced my life. She sent me this, her favorite recipe, from the Netherlands.

Preheat the oven to 350°F. Butter a medium-sized baking dish with a lid.

Arrange the potatoes and zucchini in the dish. In a small bowl, mix the sour cream, mustard, rosemary, and salt. Pour the sour cream mixture over potatoes and zucchini and mix well. Sprinkle the scallions over the potatoes, reserving 1 tablespoon for garnish. Top with grated cheese. Cover and bake for at least 45 minutes, until the potatoes are tender. Remove from the oven and garnish with the reserved scallions. Serve immediately.

4 large russet potatoes, unpeeled and thinly sliced

1 medium zucchini, sliced

½ cup sour cream

1 teaspoon prepared stone-ground mustard

2 sprigs fresh rosemary, minced (or a generous pinch of dried rosemary leaves)

Pinch of sweet paprika powder

Pinch of sea salt

3 scallions, white and green parts, minced (optional)

¾ cup grated cheddar cheese

6 to 8 dried shiitake
mushrooms

2 cups filtered water

3 tablespoons extra virgin
olive oil or sunflower oil

I large white onion, minced

½ teaspoon crushed
fenugreek seeds

4 large sweet potatoes,
peeled and cut into strips

I teaspoon garam masala
(see page 199)

I teaspoon ground
cardamom

¼ teaspoon dry-roasted
cumin seeds (see note)

¼ teaspoon ground
turmeric

½ pound firm tofu, cubed
(optional)

Soup stock or filtered water
as needed

½ cup alfalfa sprouts, for
garnish (optional)

Shiitake Mushroom Yams

SERVES 4 TO 6

In Japan, shiitake mushrooms are considerd medicine. Besides being nutritious, they contain all eight essential amino acids. They certainly make any dish taste wonderful. Enjoy this dish as a main dish with the tofu, or as a side dish without the tofu.

Soak the mushrooms in the water for 2 to 3 hours. Remove the mushrooms from the water, and reserve this water. Cut the mushrooms into thin strips with kitchen shears.

In a large cast-iron skillet or wok, warm the oil over medium heat (do not allow it to smoke). Add the onion, fenugreek seed, and mushroom strips. Stir-fry until the onion is translucent, about 2 minutes. Add the sweet potatoes, garam masala, cardamom, cumin, turmeric, and tofu. Stir until the sweet potatoes are coated with spices. Add the water that the mushrooms were soaking in. Simmer over medium heat. Watch carefully so it does not dry out and burn; add soup stock or water as needed. Continue to simmer until the sweet potatoes are tender, about 10 to 12 minutes. Garnish with alfalfa sprouts to increase the nutritional value.

Note: To roast the cumin seeds, place them in a skillet over medium-high heat. Toss them continuously in the skillet until they begin to turn a light golden color. Transfer the cumin seeds to a plate and spread them out in a single layer to cool.

Maggie's Sweet Potatoes

SERVES 4

Sweet potatoes are high in beta-carotene, and contain B vitamins, vitamin C, potassium, and iron. My Filipino lola *(grandmother) was able to keep her family from starving in exile during World War II by finding wild sweet potatoes, called* kamote *in her culture. She was a* hilot *(healer-midwife), and she taught me to encourage all expectant and breastfeeding women to eat sweet potatoes.*

This particular recipe comes from a beautiful mother named Maggie. The rosemary adds calcium to the dish, while increasing milk flow and relieving intestinal gas. Add the tofu if you plan to serve this as a main dish.

Preheat the oven to 350°F. To make the sauce, mix together the tamari, rosemary, lemon juice, and oil in a bowl. Place the sweet potatoes, onion, and tofu, if using, in a large baking dish, and toss with the sauce. Cover and bake for about 1 hour, or until the sweet potatoes are tender when pierced with a fork. Serve hot.

2 tablespoons tamari or soy sauce

1½ to 2 teaspoons rosemary leaves, fresh or dried, crushed

1 to 2 tablespoons fresh lemon juice

3 to 4 tablespoons extra virgin olive oil

4 to 5 cups cubed sweet potatoes (approximately 4 to 6 large potatoes)

1 large sweet onion (yellow or red), diced

1 pound firm tofu, cubed (optional)

4 medium beets, peeled and
cubed

4 carrots, cubed

4 russet potatoes, peeled
and cubed

2 large dill pickles, diced

2 tablespoons finely
chopped, dried or fresh
dill

½ cup extra virgin olive oil

Sea salt

Venogred Russian Vegetables

SERVES 6

*On the island of Maui, a wonderful girl once grew up. She
was invited as a teenager to represent the United States
as a youth ambassador for peace in the Soviet Union.*

*Eventually she became a mother and wrote a beautiful
book for Russian women on pregnancy, birth, and postpartum health. She is Aleshanee Akin—definitely half mother,
half angel. Here is one of the recipes she learned from her
expectant Russian sisters. This dish provides iron, potassium, niacin, copper, vitamin C, folic acid, zinc, calcium,
manganese, magnesium, and phosphorus.*

Combine the beets, carrots, and potatoes in a large pot.
Add water to cover and bring to a boil. Cook until tender
(about 15 minutes), drain, and allow the vegetables to
cool. Toss the vegetables with the pickles, dill, and oil, and
season to taste with salt. Serve warm or cold.

SOUPS

I look for any excuse to make soup—a rainy day, a snowy day, a gloomy day. When my family is under stress, I make soup. I love to make soup and bread for poetry readings and La Leche League meetings. Every "good witch" needs a few good soup recipes.

6½ cups filtered water

3 to 4 kale leaves, chopped

½ pound firm tofu, cubed

1 (½-inch) piece fresh
    ginger, peeled and thinly
    sliced

5 teaspoons miso (red or
    white)

Miso Soup

SERVES 4 TO 6

Miso is nourishing and strengthening, and the ginger aids digestion and reduces nausea. This recipe also includes tofu, which is rich in calcium. Since miso is a living food, add it only after the soup has cooled—to preserve the valuable nutrients. The perfect soup to eat if you feel a cold or flu coming on.

In a large pot, bring 6 cups of the water to a boil. Add the kale, tofu, and ginger. Decrease the heat and allow to simmer for 5 to 7 minutes. Remove from the heat and cool for 3 minutes. Meanwhile, warm the remaining ½ cup water. Mix the miso paste in the water. After the soup has cooled, gently mix in the miso mixture. Serve in bowls or heavy mugs.

Egg Drop Soup

SERVES 4 TO 6

Fresh organic eggs provide a quick source of protein. This recipe is famous for helping women who suffer from nausea and weight loss in early pregnancy.

In a large pot, bring the water, parsley, and scallion to a full boil. In a small bowl, beat the eggs until frothy and set aside. While the water is still rapidly boiling, slowly pour in the beaten eggs, while mixing gently with a fork. Remove the pot from the heat. Season to taste with tamari and serve immediately.

6 cups filtered water

I teaspoon finely chopped fresh parsley

I tablespoon finely chopped scallion, green and white parts

3 large eggs

2 to 4 teaspoons tamari or soy sauce

Déjà's Thai Soup

SERVES 6 TO 8

To say my eldest daughter, Déjà, is inventive in the kitchen is an understatement. Déjà makes food magic. This soup is a nutritious feast in itself.

Heat the oil in a large, heavy pot over medium heat. Add the chicken, shrimp, garlic, and shiitake mushrooms strips, and sauté until chicken starts to brown, about 10 minutes. Add the ginger, bok choy, and coconut milk. The curry paste is very hot, so stir in a teaspoon at a time, and taste to determine if you need to add more. Tie the lemongrass into a knot and add it to the pot. Add the lemon juice, brown sugar, fish sauce, and snow peas. Lower the heat and simmer until the chicken is cooked thoroughly and the snow peas are done but still crispy and green. Remove the lemongrass. Serve hot.

2 tablespoons toasted sesame oil

2 (6- to 8-ounce) boneless, skinless chicken breasts, cut into ½-inch pieces

½ pound medium-size shrimp, shelled and deveined

4 cloves garlic, grated

6 to 8 fresh shiitake mushroom caps, cut into strips, or dried shiitake mushrooms, revived in hot water for 30 minutes

1 (½-inch) piece fresh ginger, peeled and grated

4 cups diced bok choy

4 cups coconut milk

2 to 4 tablespoons green curry paste (available in Asian food stores)

1 stalk lemongrass (optional)

Juice of 2 lemons

¼ cup lightly packed brown sugar

¼ cup Asian fish sauce or oyster sauce (both available in Asian food stores)

¼ pound young snow peas, strings removed

Chinese Soup

SERVES 6 TO 8

The Chinese influence in the Philippines can not be under-estimated. In the Cordillera Mountains, the vegetable basket of the Philippines, we owe much of our agricultural know-how to the early Chinese immigrants to the area.

Place all of the soup ingredients in a large soup pot and bring to a boil. In a small bowl or cup, whisk together the flavor mixture ingredients. When vegetables are tender, about 10 to 12 minutes, slowly add the flavor mix. Return the soup to a boil and add the beaten egg, stirring briskly with a fork. Serve immediately.

SOUP

1 cup peeled, sliced carrots

1 cup diced celery

1 cup grated turnip

1½ cups mung bean sprouts

½ cup dried wood ear fungus (a kind of mushroom found in Asian stores) soaked for 45 minutes

¼ pound firm tofu, cubed

1 (1-inch) piece fresh ginger, peeled and grated

6 cups filtered water

FLAVOR MIXTURE

3 tablespoons soy sauce

1 tablespoon rice vinegar

2 tablespoons toasted sesame oil

1½ teaspoons powdered mustard

1 large beaten egg

12 cups filtered water

4 cups dried baby lima
   beans, washed and sorted

2 bay leaves

1 medium onion, quartered

1 onion, diced

1 tablespoon extra virgin
   olive oil

1/2 head garlic, sectioned and
   minced

4 carrots, 2 halved and 2
   sliced diagonally

6 stalks celery, 2 quartered
   and 4 diced

1/4 cup chopped fresh parsley

1 bunch kale (about 1/2
   pound), stemmed and
   torn into pieces

Pinch of sea salt

Alloysha's Baby Lima Bean Soup

SERVES 6 TO 8

This hearty soup was made by Alloysha and delivered to the home of my "daughter" Ketut, just two days before my grandson was born. What a great memory we have of Alloysha's son, Henry, and her baby, Emma, entertaining us as we waited for Ketut's baby to arrive. This soup warmed us on a rainy day in Maui.

In a large pot, combine the water, lima beans, bay leaves, quartered onion, halved carrots, and celery, and bring to a full boil. Remove from the heat and let sit for 2 hours.

Heat the oil in a large, heavy saucepan over medium heat. Add the diced onion and sauté until translucent, about 1 minute. Add the garlic and sliced carrots, and continue to sauté for 3 to 5 minutes until garlic starts to brown. Add the diced celery, parsley, and kale, and sauté for an additional 5 minutes. Remove from the heat. Add the vegetable mixture to the pot of lima beans and bring to a boil. Add salt to taste. Decrease the heat and simmer until the lima beans are tender and fully cooked, about 1 hour.

Lemon Lentil Soup

SERVES 6 TO 8

When the Saint Ammachi came to give darshan *(hugs of healing love and compassion) in Mt. Pleasant, Iowa, I was blessed to meet Karen Kellogg. Karen shared this, her wonderful lemon lentil soup recipe. The first time I tested Karen's recipe, two families I had caught babies for dropped by. One whiff of the soup cooking in the pot, and they all stayed for diner. Everyone enjoyed two big bowls. Namaste, Karen.*

Heat ⅓ cup of the oil in large deep saucepan over medium heat. Add the onion and cook, stirring, until soft, about 10 minutes. Add the cinnamon, lentils, and ginger, and cook for 10 to 15 minutes more, stirring often. Add the stock, boiling water, and the cayenne, and bring to a boil. Decrease the heat to low and simmer for 20 minutes, until the lentils are completely soft. Add the lemon juice, zest, and pulp and season to taste with salt. Cook for an additional 15 minutes to allow the flavors to blend.

In a small pan, heat the remaining 1 tablespoon of oil and add the onion and garlic. Sauté over medium heat for 1 to 2 minutes until golden brown, then add to the soup. Garnish the soup with the chopped cilantro and serve.

⅓ cup plus 1 tablespoon extra virgin olive oil

1 onion, thinly sliced

2 cinnamon sticks

2 cups red lentils, washed

1 (1-inch) piece fresh ginger, peeled and grated

8 cups vegetable or chicken broth

2½ cups filtered water, boiling

¼ teaspoon cayenne pepper

1 lemon: juice, grated zest, and pulp

Sea salt

1 small onion, diced

1 clove garlic, chopped

1 bunch cilantro, stewed and chopped, for garnish

6 cups filtered water

3 beets, peeled and cut into
$\frac{1}{2}$-inch cubes

2 gabi roots (see Note) or
russet potatoes, peeled
and cut into $\frac{1}{2}$-inch cubes

3 cloves garlic

1 onion, diced

1 teaspoon curry powder

1 tablespoon sea salt

$\frac{1}{2}$ pound firm tofu, cut into
$\frac{1}{2}$-inch cubes

1 small handful of fresh
cilantro leaves, chopped,
for garnish

Sesame Gomashio, for
garnish (see page 198)

Cream of Beet Soup

SERVES 4 TO 6

*Beets and tofu are both touted as being high in calcium.
Pregnant and breastfeeding women, and those of us who
admit to being middle-aged, must get plenty of calcium for
the health of our bones and teeth. This creamy soup contains no dairy and you won't miss it.*

In a large soup pot, combine the water, beets, gabi, garlic,
onion, curry and salt, and bring to a boil. When the beets
are half cooked, about 5 to 6 minutes, add the tofu.
Decrease the heat and simmer. Once the gabi and beets are
well-cooked, about 10 to 15 more minutes, pour half of
the soup into the blender and blend until smooth and
creamy. Transfer the blended soup to another pot, and
blend the second half of the soup mixture. Combine the
blended mixtures and serve in bowls garnished with fresh
cilantro and gomashio.

Note: Gabi root is a hairy root vegetable, with a very rough
appearance. Its taste is starchy with a unique flavor all its
own. Store gabi root as you would any potato, and peel
before cutting to remove rough outer appearance. It can be
found in Asian or whole foods stores.

Cream of Broccoli Soup

SERVES 6 TO 8

Broccoli is one of those vegetables that just calls out to me when I spot it in the market. Perhaps it's the irresistible deep green that makes me want to take it home. The tofu in this recipe provides calcium and protein. Broccoli has been found to fight cancer, so it's not just delicious food—it is medicine as well.

In a medium pot, steam the broccoli in water until tender, about 4 to 5 minutes. Heat the oil in a large, heavy saucepan over medium heat. Add the garlic, leek, mushrooms, and rosemary, and sauté for about 3 minutes until garlic is getting golden. Place the broccoli in a food processor or blender with the tofu and water and process until creamy. Pour the broccoli mixture back into the pot and reheat. Add the sautéed ingredients and salt to taste. Stir until well mixed and serve.

1½ pounds fresh broccoli, stems peeled, stems and tops cut into 1- to 2-inch pieces

2 tablespoons extra virgin olive oil

4 cloves garlic, crushed

1 large leek, white part only, rinsed well and sliced

½ pound button mushrooms, sliced

¼ teaspoon fresh or dried rosemary, crushed

½ pound firm tofu, cubed

6 cups filtered water

Sea salt

1 tablespoon toasted sesame oil

4 to 5 cloves garlic, minced

1 small red onion, diced

6 cups filtered water

1 teaspoon wasabi powder

1 pound russet potatoes, washed and diced

1 handful (approximately 2 to 3 ounces) dried Hijiki seaweed, crumbled

1 tablespoon red miso

Freshly ground black pepper

Potato Hijiki Soup

SERVES 4 TO 6

This is a mineral-rich soup, perfect for alleviating those winter aches and pains. Hijiki seaweed (available in most health-food stores) is especially good for promoting healthy organs and strong, shiny hair. This sea vegetable is 10–20% protein and is high in fiber. Enjoy!

In a large saucepan, heat the oil over medium heat. Add the garlic and onion and sauté until golden brown. Add the water and bring the mixture to a boil. In a small bowl, dissolve the wasabi in a little warm water and add to the soup. Add the potatoes and seaweed. Cook until potatoes are tender and well done, about 10 to 13 minutes. Remove ⅔ cup of the broth from the pot and let it cool for five minutes, then add the miso to this broth. Mix with a fork until the miso is thoroughly dissolved. Turn off the heat under the soup pot and allow the soup to cool for 5 minutes. Slowly add the miso/broth mixture. Season to taste with pepper and serve.

Pumpkin Soup

SERVES 4 TO 6

In Japan, shiitake mushrooms and ginger are known to have healing powers. This soup will warm your bones and soothe your spirits.

Soak the shiitake mushrooms for 1 hour or more in the water. Save the mushroom water to make the soup. With kitchen shears or a paring knife, cut the softened mushrooms into strips.

In a large pot, combine the mushroom water, mushrooms, pumpkin, and ginger and bring to a boil. Lower the heat and simmer until pumpkin is easily mashed (about 20 to 25 minutes), mashing the pumpkin by using a potato masher right in the cooking pot. Add the coconut milk and salt to taste. Serve steaming hot with gomashio on top.

6 to 8 dried shiitake mushrooms

4 cups filtered water

1 small pumpkin or acorn squash (approximately 1 to 1½ pounds), peeled, seeded, and cubed

1 (1-inch) piece fresh ginger, peeled and grated

1 cup coconut milk

Sea salt

Sesame Gomashio (see page 198), for garnish

¾ cup raw cashew nuts

2 cups filtered water

I small pumpkin (I to I½ pounds), peeled, seeded, and cubed

2 cups vegetable stock

I cinnamon stick

Sea salt

½ bunch cilantro, stemmed, for garnish

Cashew Pumpkin Soup

SERVES 4 TO 6

With its delicious cinnamon flavor, this creamy nondairy soup is a real child pleaser. It also helps alleviate pregnancy nausea and aids in digestion.

Soak the cashews in the water for 2 hours or longer (overnight in the refrigerator is okay).

In a large pot, combine the pumpkin with the vegetable stock and bring to a boil. Add the cinnamon stick and cook until the pumpkin falls apart when stirred, about 20 to 25 minutes.

In the blender, puree the cashews with their soaking water until creamy. Add to the cooked pumpkin and salt to taste. Remove the cinnamon stick before serving and garnish generously with cilantro.

Sinigang

SERVES 6

This high-protein Filipino stand-by is one of my favorites. My lola *was the very most talented sinigang-maker on the planet; the second best was my mother. You may try this recipe with any number of freshwater or saltwater fish. Experiment to find your favorite.*

Bring the water to a boil in a large pot. Add the garlic, ginger, and sweet potatoes. Decrease the heat and simmer until the sweet potatoes are nearly done, about 10 to 15 minutes. Add the bok choy, tomato, fish sauce, and fresh fish. Cover and continue to simmer until the fish is cooked through, about 5 to 7 minutes. Season to taste with pepper and serve.

10 cups filtered water

2 cloves garlic, crushed

1 (2-inch) piece fresh ginger, peeled and thinly sliced

2 sweet potatoes, peeled and cubed

1/3 pound bok choy, chopped into bite-sized pieces

1 medium tomato, diced

1/4 cup Asian fish sauce (found in whole-foods and Asian stores) or 1/4 cup tamari

1/2 pound fresh fish fillet, cut into 2- to 3-inch pieces

Freshly ground black pepper

Soups from the Philippine Mountains

*H*igh in the Cordillera Mountains of Luzon lies the summer capital of the Philippines, Baguio City, my mother's hometown. In Baguio we enjoy clear sunny days, and sometimes the nights are quite chilly. During the rainy season, we close up our houses against the typhoon winds. *"Naglammin,"* we say in Ilokano, when it's cold outside. Many homes still have beautiful crude wood-fire stoves built into the corner of the ground floor. From these fires the aroma of a hearty soup warms the Filipino home and the heart.

2 tablespoons extra virgin
   olive oil

4 large ripe tomatoes,
   blanched and peeled (see
   Note) or 1 medium can
   peeled tomatoes

1 medium zucchini, cut into
   bite-sized pieces

1 green bell pepper, seeded
   and cut into bite-sized
   pieces

1 head broccoli, stems
   peeled and stem and top
   cut into bite-sized pieces

1 block (10 to 12 ounces) firm
   tofu, cubed or crumbled

1 teaspoon dried or fresh dill
   weed plus 1/2 teaspoon,
   chopped, for garnish

1/2 teaspoon tarragon

1 teaspoon sea salt

Rainy Day Tomato Soup

SERVES 6 TO 8

This creamy, dairy-free soup is quick and loaded with calcium, protein, vitamins, and minerals. It's a good pick-me-up on a gloomy day.

Heat the oil in a large, heavy saucepan over medium heat. Add the tomatoes, zucchini, green pepper, and broccoli and sauté for 3 to 5 minutes, until the vegetables become soft.

Combine the tofu, dill, tarragon, and salt in a food processor or blender and process until smooth. Using a slotted spoon to reserve the vegetable stock in the pot, add the vegetables to the food processor and blend again. Pour the blended mixture back into the pot with the reserved stock, and cook over low heat for 7 to 10 minutes. Serve with a sprinkling of dill.

Note: To blanch and peel the tomatoes, fill a large bowl with water and ice cubes. Bring a large pot of water to a boil. Remove the cores from the tomatoes and using a fork, plunge each one into boiling water for 10 seconds, then into the iced water to cool. Peel the skin and cut each tomato into four wedges.

Arroz Caldo

SERVES 6 TO 8

Arroz caldo is a healing Filipino chicken soup. A version of this recipe is popular in Indonesia, where it is called bur-bur Ayam. On gloomy, rainy days in the mountain city of Baguio, where my mother was born and raised, one could always find a makeshift corner café that sold steaming bowls of arroz caldo. This "chicken soup for the Filipino soul" costs only a few centavos when you buy it on the street. It is so nourishing that I make it at home during cold and flu season.

Heat the oil in a large, deep pot over medium-high heat. Add the chicken, garlic, and ginger, and sauté until the chicken begins to brown. Add the rice to the chicken, and stir well. Add the boiling water along with the carrots. Cover and bring the mixture to a boil, then lower the heat, and simmer for 1 hour, until it all becomes a lovely porridge. Check occasionally to ensure there is plenty of liquid. If the porridge appears dry, add water. Season to taste with salt and garnish with fresh cilantro. Serve hot.

¼ cup extra virgin olive oil

1 pound chicken, skinned and cut into bite-size pieces

2 to 4 cloves garlic, crushed

2 to 3 inches fresh ginger, peeled, cut into 1-inch sections, and crushed

1 cup uncooked brown rice, soaked in filtered water for 1 hour or more

6 cups filtered water, boiling

3 carrots, sliced into ½-inch rounds

Sea salt

¼ cup chopped fresh cilantro, for garnish

ENTRÉES

As a busy mom you will want to have a few main-course recipes under your belt. These should be for practical dishes that are easy to prepare and use ingredients with which you are familiar. I call them my standbys, as I can always whip them up in a pinch. The entrées in this chapter are favorites from my friends and family.

Tahini Stir-Fry

SERVES 4

3 to 4 tablespoons extra virgin olive oil

1 (1-inch) piece ginger root, peeled and grated

1 onion, diced (optional)

2 to 3 cloves garlic, minced (optional)

Approximately 6 cups fresh veggies cut into bite-size pieces, such as broccoli, cauliflower, zucchini, carrots, sweet potatoes, russet potatoes, snap peas, green beans, Brussels sprouts, or leafy greens

1/3 cup filtered water or milk, plus more as needed

2 tablespoons tamari or soy sauce

1/2 cup sesame tahini

1/3 cup filtered water

This main dish can even be served as breakfast. It is made with sesame tahini, which makes it rich in calcium, protein, vitamins A and E, zinc, copper, magnesium, phosphorus, iron, and potassium. In the Middle East, sesame is called the "seed of immortality." You can use any vegetables you happen to have in your garden or larder. When unexpected guests arrive hungry, this is easy and fun to whip up. Serve by itself, over rice, or even over toast.

Heat the oil in a wok or large saucepan over medium heat. Add the ginger, onion, and garlic, and sauté for 1 minute until the onion becomes translucent. Add the vegetables that take longer to cook, such as the potatoes, broccoli, cauliflower, and carrots. Add a little water or milk and cover. Allow the vegetables to steam for 3 to 5 minutes. Add the faster-cooking veggies, such as the peas and green beans. Leafy greens should be added last. Splash the tamari over all, add more water/milk as needed, cover and allow to steam until veggies are done, but still bright in color, about 5 to 7 more minutes.

Meanwhile, combine the tahini with 1/3 cup water in a small bowl, and mix until smooth. Turn off the heat under the veggies and drizzle the tahini sauce over all. Replace the cover and let sit for a couple of minutes. Serve hot.

Tofu Chop Chay

SERVES 6

Chop chay is a standard entrée in Indonesia. This version is protein- and calcium-rich, due to the inclusion of tofu. Serve over rice or the grain of your choice.

Heat the oils in a wok or large, heavy saucepan over medium heat. Add the carrots, onion, cabbage, kale, and tofu, and sauté for 5 to 7 minutes until the onion becomes translucent. Add ½ cup of the water, cover, and let simmer on low heat until the vegetables are tender, but still colorful.

To make the sauce, whisk together the tamari, cornstarch, and remaining ½ cup of water in a small bowl until thoroughly blended. When the vegetables are tender, add the sauce. Cover and simmer for 2 more minutes, until the sauce is translucent. Serve hot.

- 1 tablespoon extra virgin olive oil
- 1 teaspoon toasted sesame oil
- 2 carrots, thinly sliced
- 1 small red onion, diced
- ½ head green cabbage, cored and chopped
- 1 bunch kale, stemmed and chopped
- 1 pound firm tofu
- 1 cup filtered water
- 1½ tablespoons tamari or soy sauce
- 1 tablespoon cornstarch

FALAFEL BALLS

3 cups dried garbanzo beans

1 bunch parsley, stemmed
   and chopped

5 to 6 cloves garlic, chopped

¼ cup fresh lemon juice

Salt

Olive oil, for frying

TAHINI SAUCE

1 cup sesame tahini

1½ to 2 cups filtered water

Juice of 1½ lemons

Sea salt

SALAD

1 head leafy lettuce, finely
   chopped

2 tomatoes, cored and diced

3 kosher dill pickles, diced

Black kalmata olives, pitted
   (optional)

Feta cheese, crumbled
   (optional)

Cucumber Raita (page 88)
   (optional)

2 packages pita bread
   (hearty whole-grain pitas
   are recommended)

Additional lettuce, for
   garnish

Marie's Falafel

SERVES 8 OR MORE

When I was a teenager I worked at Uncle Mustache Falafel in Isla Vista, California. I learned to make a fantastic falafel sandwich, but never found out the secret of how to make the excellent falafel ball mix, until my dear friend Marie Zenack shared her recipe with me. The sauce is also important. My boss at Uncle Mustache, Abdul, would say, "It should be so saucy that the customer has to bite and suck when eating our falafel." Marie taught me that the garbanzo beans must be sprouted first, so they will be a living food. This traditional Middle Eastern dish is a hearty complete meal. Our family enjoys falafel so much that when we make it, we invite several friends over to share our feast.

Soak the beans in a large bowl in at least 8 cups water for 1 to 2 days, changing the water every few hours. When your kitchen is quiet, as in the middle of the night, you may hear the garbanzos popping open, as the water activates the life force stored within each bean. It is very important to remember to change the water every few hours.

After the beans have soaked and sprouted, grind them along with the parsley, garlic, lemon juice and salt (to taste) in a food processor or powerful blender. You will have to do the grinding in batches. Process or blend until the falafel ball mix looks like a coarse wet meal.

Preheat the oven to 200°F. To prepare the falafel balls, heat 1½ to 2 inches of oil in a wok or a small cast-iron skillet. When the oil is hot but not smoking, form falafel balls by using a tablespoon to scoop mix, compress a bit with your palm and carefully, slowly, lower gently into the hot oil. If you do it just right the balls will hold together.

Fry a half dozen or so at a time, until golden brown, turning once with a fork. The balls should be crispy on the outside and raw (alive) on the inside. Remove the balls from the oil with a slotted spoon and transfer them onto paper towel-lined plates to drain. Place the falafel balls in the warm oven until you are ready to serve. Continue making more falafel balls until all the mix is used.

To make the tahini sauce, combine the tahini, 1½ cups water, lemon juice, and salt (to taste) in a medium bowl. Either using a mixer or by hand, combine the ingredients until smooth and creamy. The sauce should be the consistency of thick cream, viscous but thin enough to be poured. Add the additional ½ cup water in small increments to make a thinner sauce.

To make the salad, combine the lettuce, tomatoes, and pickles in a medium bowl. Add the olives, feta cheese, and/or raita. Toss to mix and set aside.

To assemble the falafels, warm the pita bread in the oven two at a time. Slice just a thin crescent away from one side of the bread. Squeeze it gently, so it will open (this works well when the bread is warmed, but don't let it get hard in the oven). Holding the bread so it is gaping open, place a thin layer of the salad mixture inside. Follow with about four falafel balls, and then another layer of salad mixture. Make the layers thin, so as not to overstuff the falafel. Hold the sandwich upright and drizzle 3 to 5 tablespoons of tahini sauce into it. Top the opening of the falafel sandwich with a garnish of lettuce, and a bit of tomato, pickle, or olive.

Vegetables

2 tablespoons extra virgin olive oil or ghee (see page 198)

2 carrots, thinly sliced

1 stalk broccoli, stem peeled, stem and top cut into bite-size pieces

1 medium sized zucchini, sliced

Filling

8 ounces tempeh, cubed

½ pound firm tofu, cubed

Sauce

¼ cup sunflower seed butter (available at most natural food stores)

2 cups soy milk

3 tablespoons extra virgin olive oil

Pinch of ground coriander

Pinch of ground fennel seeds

Pinch of ground turmeric

Pinch of freshly ground black pepper

Salt

1 teaspoon fresh lemon juice

1 package 10-inch whole wheat tortillas or chapati

Veggie Wraps with Sunflower Butter Sauce

SERVES 4 TO 6

Alesia, mother of Charan and Chay-chay, advises moms to use only the best organic ingredients. This colorful medly of vitamin-rich ingredients is topped off with a calcium- and protein-rich sauce.

To make the vegetables, heat 1½ tablespoons of the oil in a wok or large cast-iron skillet over medium heat. Add the carrots and broccoli, and sauté for 2 to 3 minutes until about half-cooked. Add the zucchini and continue to sauté for an additional 2 to 3 minutes. The vegetables are ready when tender. In a separate pan, over medium heat, heat remaining oil and sauté tempeh and tofu until golden brown, about 5 minutes.

To make the sauce, heat a small saucepan over medium-low heat. Add the sunflower seed butter and soy milk, and whisk together until mixture is smooth. Stir in the olive oil, coriander, fennel, turmeric, and pepper, and salt to taste. Turn off the heat, add the lemon juice, and stir.

To assemble the wraps, warm the tortillas or chapattis over medium heat in a dry cast-iron skillet. Spoon the vegetables onto tortillas, then spoon the filling onto the vegetable mix. Squeeze a bit of lemon over the mixture and drizzle the sauce on top. Wrap, eat, and enjoy!

Creamy Sweet Potatoes with Tempeh

SERVES 4 TO 6

Sweet potatoes are so good for our reproductive organs that I believe they are medicine. This dairy-free recipe is creamy and delicious. It is fantastic with Bruce's Bachelor Rice (see page 166).

Heat the oil in a large cast-iron skillet with a tight-fitting lid over medium heat. Add the sweet potatoes, onion, tempeh, and ginger, and sauté until the onions are translucent, about 4 to 5 minutes, stirring often. Add the water and bring to a boil. Decrease the heat to a simmer and cover. Check every few minutes. When the sweet potatoes are just getting tender, about 8 to 10 minutes, add the coconut milk and salt, and stir. Add the snow peas, cover, and allow to cook until peas are just done, but still bright green and slightly crisp, about 3 to 4 minutes. Serve hot.

3 tablespoons toasted sesame oil

2 to 3 large sweet potatoes, washed and cubed

1 onion, diced

8 ounces tempeh (or substitute firm tofu), cubed

1 (1½-inch) piece fresh ginger, peeled and grated

½ cup filtered water

1 cup coconut milk

1½ teaspoons sea salt

½ pound snow peas, trimmed

1 pound whole-grain egg
   noodles

Extra virgin olive oil, plus 2
   tablespoons for the sauce

8 ounces firm tofu, cubed

2 stalks celery, diced

1 green bell pepper, seeded
   and chopped

1 tablespoon tamari or soy
   sauce

1 teaspoon fresh or dried dill
   weed

$\frac{1}{2}$ teaspoon ground
   coriander

1 teaspoon fresh oregano

$\frac{1}{2}$ cup fresh basil leaves

Pinch of freshly ground
   black pepper

Pinch of sea salt

2 tablespoons vegetarian
   protein powder (available
   in health-food stores)

$\frac{3}{4}$ cup filtered water

1 cup sour cream

1 tablespoon organic white
   or whole wheat flour

$\frac{1}{2}$ cup pitted kalmata olives
   (optional)

Marci's Tofu Stroganoff

SERVES 6

Marci has been such a blessing. She's a doula (a woman who mothers the mother during birth and postpartum) and has accompanied me to many wonderful births. Her loving touch is evident in this protein-rich entrée.

Cook the noodles in plenty of boiling salted water following the directions on package, or until al dente. Drain, and drizzle in a little olive oil so the noodles don't stick together.

While the noodles are cooking, heat 1 tablespoon of the oil in a wok or large saucepan over medium heat. Add the tofu and sauté until it begins to brown, about 4 minutes. Add the celery, green pepper, tamari, spices, and remaining tablespoon of olive oil, and continue to sauté until the vegetables are half cooked, about 3 to 4 minutes.

In a small bowl, whisk together the protein powder and water. Add to the tofu mixture and simmer for 20 minutes.

Blend together the sour cream and the flour and add to the tofu mixture. Add the olives. Continue to simmer while stirring, until the mixture is thick and well blended, about 5 to 6 minutes.

To serve, place the noodles in a large serving bowl. Pour the thickened tofu and veggie mixture over the noodles and toss together.

Italian Tofu

SERVES 4 TO 6

This is a quick and satisfying dish. It was invented when our oven was broken, and we were craving lasagna.

Heat the oil in a wok or large saucepan over medium heat. Add the onions, chard, tofu, oregano, basil, and salt, and sauté for 45 minutes, until onions are translucent and tofu begins to brown, stirring occasionally. Add the tomato sauce, dot with spoonfuls of the ricotta cheese, and sprinkle with the Parmesan cheese. Cover, decrease the heat, and allow to simmer for 15 to 20 minutes, until the chard is completely tender and the flavors are well blended.

Meanwhile, to cook the pasta, bring 4 quarts of water and 1 teaspoon salt to a rapid boil. Add the pasta and cook, uncovered, stirring frequently, until pasta is al dente. Rigatoni takes 13 to 15 minutes; rotini, 9 to 11 minutes; and thin spaghetti, 7 to 9 minutes. Drain well. Toss olive oil over pasta. Serve the pasta and the Italian tofu in their own serving bowls so folks can take as little or as much of each, as they like.

2 tablespoons extra virgin olive oil

2 onions, diced

1 bunch Swiss chard (about ¾ pound), finely chopped

1½ pounds firm tofu, cubed

1 teaspoon chopped fresh oregano

1 teaspoon chopped fresh basil

Pinch of sea salt

1 (28-ounce) can plain tomato sauce

1 pound ricotta cheese

¼ cup grated Parmesan cheese

1 pound pasta, such as rigatoni, rotini, or thin spaghetti

1 teaspoon salt for cooking pasta

3 tablespoons extra virgin olive oil for pasta

2 tablespoons toasted
   sesame oil

8 ounces tempeh, cut into
   bite-size pieces

1 yellow onion, diced

1 red bell pepper, seeded and
   diced

1 tablespoon apple cider
   vinegar

1 tablespoon tamari or soy
   sauce

¼ cup filtered water

¼ pound endive, chopped (or
   substitute kale or extra
   chard)

¼ pound Swiss chard,
   chopped

Tempeh à la Wil

SERVES 4

While I was pregnant I discovered that my husband can really cook. He always made sure I was comfortable and well-fed. Tempeh is made with soybeans and is a good source of protein while being low in saturated fat. It is commonly available in natural food stores. The colorful vegetables in this dish just shout vitamins and minerals! This dish is wonderful served over any grain, especially Quinoa and Brown Rice (page 165).

Heat the oil in a wok or large cast-iron skillet with a lid over medium heat. Add the tempeh and onion and sauté until the tempeh begins to brown and the onion is translucent, about 10 to 15 minutes. Add the bell pepper and sauté for 1 minute more.

In a small bowl, mix together the vinegar, tamari, and water. Toss the endive and chard into the skillet, pour the tamari mixture over it, and cover. When the wok begins to steam, decrease the heat, and steam the green vegetables until they are just cooked, but still firm and full of color, about 3 to 4 minutes. Serve hot.

Lumpia
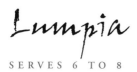

SERVES 6 TO 8

The best lumpias in this world are made by my mother. The second best can be found only in Baguio City, at the street vendor's stall between the Empire Theater and the 50s Café. Usually I make them vegetarian, but I offer a chicken version, too.

To make the filling, stir the tamari and cornstarch together in a medium bowl. Add the tofu or chicken and toss to coat.

Heat the sesame oil in a wok or large skillet over medium-high heat. Do not let it smoke. Stir-fry the tofu mixture. Add the carrots, onion, garlic, and ginger. Keep stirring until the onions are translucent and the chicken is cooked through, about 10 to 15 minutes. Add the mung beans and continue to stir-fry for about 3 more minutes. Set aside to cool for 15 minutes.

To assemble the lumpias, place one wrapper on a tray or plate. Place 1½ to 2 tablespoons of filling in the center of the wrapper. Firmly roll halfway. Using a bit of water, moisten the remaining edges of the wrapper. Tuck the sides over and roll the rest of the way, sealing the moist edges. At this point, you may wrap and freeze the lumpias for later use. Allow frozen lumpias to thaw for 20 to 30 minutes before frying, following the directions below.

To fry the lumpias, heat the olive oil, about 1½ to 2 inches of it, in a wok or heavy frying pan to about 375° F. Carefully place a few lumpias into the heated oil, and fry them until golden brown, about 3 minutes, turning once. Drain well before serving.

To make the sauce, mix all the sauce ingredients together in saucepan and heat over medium heat, stirring constantly as it thickens. Serve warm with the lumpias.

FILLING

¼ cup tamari or soy sauce

I teaspoon cornstarch

I pound firm tofu, diced, and/or 2 boneless chicken breasts, skinned and diced

2 tablespoons toasted sesame oil

2 carrots, grated

I onion, diced

I (1-inch) piece fresh ginger, grated

2 cloves garlic, minced

I pound mung bean sprouts

I package egg roll wrappers (about 20 per package)

Olive oil, for frying

SAUCE

¼ cup tamari or soy sauce

2 teaspoons cornstarch

¼ cup filtered water

¼ cup apple cider or rice vinegar

I teaspoon fresh lemon juice

¼ teaspoon ground ginger

½ teaspoon raw sugar or sucanat

2 tablespoons extra virgin olive oil

I pound Swiss chard or kale, stemmed and finely chopped

I onion, finely diced

4 cloves garlic, minced (optional)

Sea salt

¼ cup filtered water

I pound ricotta cheese

½ pound feta cheese, crumbled

¼ teaspoon freshly grated nutmeg

¼ cup pitted kalmata olives, diced

½ cup chopped pecans (optional)

½ cup (I stick) butter

½ (16-ounce) package filo dough, thawed if frozen

Pinch of sweet paprika

¼ cup grated Parmesan cheese

Beccita's Delight

SERVES 6 TO 8

When Rebecca, better known as "Beccita," came with her husband, Scott, and daughter, Surreal, to live beside us and birth her baby Inti, this dish was invented. It began with an opportunity to get a case of frozen organic whole-wheat filo dough at a bargain price from our food co-op. That was just before Inti's birth. During Beccita's postpartum days, both families feasted on this dish many times, and we never got tired of it. One 16-ounce package of filo dough is enough to make this dish and Surreal's Delight for dessert (page 229), so we always made them together, just as Beccita and Surreal are always together!

Preheat the oven to 350°F.

To make the filling, heat the oil in a wok or large saucepan over medium heat. Add the chard and onion and sauté for 3 to 5 minutes. Add the garlic, salt to taste, and sauté for an additional 3 minutes. Add the water, cover, and allow to steam for 3 to 5 minutes, until vegetables are partly cooked and still bright green.

In a large bowl, mix the ricotta cheese with the feta, nutmeg, olives, and pecans. Add the cooked, drained vegetables and mix well.

To assemble, melt the butter in a small saucepan over very low heat. Using a pastry brush, lightly coat the bottom of a 9-by-13-by-2-inch glass or enamel baking pan with butter. Working quickly so the filo dough doesn't dry out, unroll the dough and loosely cover with a damp (not wet) cloth or damp paper towels to keep it from drying out as you work. Lay a sheet of filo in the dish as neatly and flat as possible. Fold the filo sheet in half widthwise to make it fit in the pan. Brush with butter. Repeat this step with three sheets of filo, brushing with butter between each sheet. After the fourth sheet of filo has been placed in the baking pan, spoon half of the filling mixture on top, spreading it out evenly. Lay another filo sheet on top of the mixture, brush it with butter, and fold. Repeat this step with three sheets of filo, brushing with butter between each sheet. Spoon the other half of the filling on top. Lay another filo sheet on top of the mixture, brush it with butter, and fold. Repeat this step with two sheets of filo, brushing with butter between each sheet. Before placing the final layer of filo dough, sprinkle with the Parmesan cheese. After you brush the top layer of filo with butter, dust it with paprika. Before baking, score the top layer of filo into serving-size portions.

Bake for about 45 minutes to 1 hour or until the top is golden brown. Allow to cool for 10 minutes before serving.

- 4 bunches (about ¾ pound each) Swiss chard, stemmed and chopped
- 4 bunches (about ¾ pound each) spinach, stemmed and chopped
- 8 ounces soft silken tofu
- 2 cups grated Romano or Parmesan cheese
- 2 tablespoons arrowroot powder
- 1 teaspoon freshly grated nutmeg
- 2 dashes ume plum vinegar or tamari or more to taste
- ¼ teaspoon freshly ground black pepper
- 8 ounces feta cheese, crumbled
- ½ bunch parsley, stemmed and finely chopped

- ¾ to 1 cup (1½ to 2 sticks) unsalted butter, melted
- 2 (16 ounce) packages whole-wheat filo dough, thawed if frozen

Christina's Spanikopita

SERVES 16

Our daughter Lakota admires her friend Christina for good reason; she's a wonderful mother. Her home is warm and well lived in, with evidence of her three children's homeschooling projects all over the place. In the dead of winter, you'll find Christina in the kitchen with the children, the wood stove blazing, all of them dressed for the beach. She is coziness incarnate. Her recipe is an organic blend of nutritious and delicious. You'll need to plan ahead when making this dish, as it must be refrigerated for 2 hours before baking.

Steam the greens for 3 to 4 minutes, set aside to cool, and drain excess water.

To make the filling, place the tofu in a large bowl and stir with a wooden spoon until smooth. Add the Romano cheese, arrowroot, nutmeg, vinegar, and pepper. Taste to check the seasoning; if the tofu flavor comes through too strongly, add a dash or two more of the vinegar. Add the feta cheese, parsley, and the steamed greens. Cover with plastic wrap and place in the refrigerator until you are ready to use it.

To assemble melt the butter in a small saucepan over low heat. Using a pastry brush, lightly coat the bottom of two 9-by-13-inch glass or enamel baking pans with the butter. Working quickly so the filo doesn't dry out, unroll the filo dough from one box and cut the entire stack into halves, so the sheets will fit your baking dishes (lying crosswise). Loosely cover the filo dough with a damp (not wet) cloth or damp paper towels to keep it from drying out as you work.

Place a sheet of filo dough in a pan and brush lightly with butter. Repeat until half of the package of filo dough is used. Use the other half package to line the second baking pan. Don't worry about getting every bit of each sheet of filo covered with butter—until you get to the last two sheets.

Divide the filling equally between the two pans. Spread it out evenly and carefully over the stacked, buttered filo dough.

Open the second package of filo dough. Unroll it and cut the entire stack into halves, just as you did the first package. Place a sheet of filo over the filling, brush lightly with melted butter, and repeat. Use half of the package of filo dough on each pan of spanikopita. Make sure the last two layers of filo in each pan are thoroughly covered with melted butter. Cover and refrigerate for 2 hours or overnight.

Preheat the oven to 350°F. Before baking, score the top layer of filo into serving-size portions. Bake, uncovered, for 45 minutes to 1 hour, until the top is golden brown. Allow the dish to cool for 10 minutes before slicing and serving.

Notes for Busy Moms

- Spanikopita can be frozen before baking. Take it out the night before you want to eat it and put it in your refrigerator to defrost. Bake as described at left.
- This dish is very labor-intensive. However, you can spread out the process over several days like this:

Day 1: Wash, steam, and dry the greens. Refrigerate.

Day 2: Prepare filling and refrigerate.

Day 3: Assemble spanikopita and refrigerate (or freeze) until you are ready to bake. (My children like to "paint" the butter on the layers of filo.)

2 tablespoons extra virgin
olive oil

2 bunches Swiss chard,
chopped

I bunch kale, stemmed and
chopped

I clove garlic, grated

5 large eggs

3 tablespoons Dijon
mustard

I tablespoon sherry

½ pound Monterey Jack
cheese, grated

Unbaked pie shell (see page
223)

Plain yogurt, for garnish
(optional)

Christine's Dijon Green Quiche

SERVES 6 TO 8

What an honor it was to be present for the birth of Christine's and Dean's fourth daughter, Olivia. This baby, born at home in a tub of water, floated sweetly into her father's arms. Christine, the picture of health and beauty, was completely focused and centered as she brought her baby Earth-side. This recipe is as French as Christine, who makes it for their wonderful restaurant, The Crepe Escape. She and Dean use only the finest organic ingredients and grow the vegetables in their greenhouse year-round. Serve with a mixed green salad on the side.

Preheat the oven to 375°F.

Heat the oil in a wok or a large, heavy saucepan. Add the chard, kale, and garlic, and sauté until the greens are cooked, but still firm and full of color—about 7 to 10 minutes. Remove from the heat.

In a medium bowl, beat the eggs with the mustard and sherry. Add the cheese and mix well. Pour the egg mixture into the greens and mix well. Pour the filling mix into the pie shell.

Bake for 35 to 40 minutes, until the crust is golden brown and a knife inserted in the center comes out clean.

Cut into 6 to 8 wedges and serve warm. Top each serving with a dollop of plain yogurt for extra calcium.

Santa Fe Quiche

SERVES 6 TO 8

This delicious quiche recipe also comes to you by way of Christine Goodale, my favorite French chef.

Preheat the oven to 375°F.

Heat the oil in a wok or a large, heavy saucepan over medium heat. Add the onion, bell pepper, garlic, and chili powder, and sauté until the onion is soft, 3 to 4 minutes. Add the tomatoes, corn, and olives and continue to sauté for an additional 3 minutes; the tomatoes will be about cooked. Decrease the heat and simmer.

In a medium bowl, beat together the eggs and cheese. Pour the vegetable mixture into the pie shell, then pour egg and cheese mixture over all.

Bake for 35 to 40 minutes, or until the crust is golden brown and a knife inserted in the center comes out clean.

Cut into 6 to 8 wedges and serve warm with a dollop of sour cream on top of each serving.

1 tablespoon extra virgin olive oil

1/2 onion, diced

1 green bell pepper, seeded and diced

1 clove minced garlic

1 tablespoon chili powder

1 cup diced fresh tomatoes

1 can corn

1 can sliced black olives

4 large eggs

1/2 pound Monterey Jack cheese, grated

Unbaked pie shell (see page 223)

Sour cream, as garnish

1 tablespoon extra virgin
   olive oil
⅓ pound arugula, stemmed
   and coarsely chopped

4 large eggs
2 cups cow's or goat's milk
¼ cup grated Parmesan
   cheese
½ cup black kalmata olives,
   pitted and diced
Freshly grated nutmeg

Unbaked pie shell (see page
   223)

Olive–Arugula Quiche

SERVES 6 TO 8

Some people (like me) just love bitter vegetables. Arugula definitely falls into this category. This protein-rich dish is also packed with vitamins and minerals.

Preheat the oven to 375°F.

Heat the oil in a wok or large, heavy saucepan over medium heat. Add the arugula and sauté until soft, 5 to 6 minutes.

In a deep, medium-sized bowl, beat the eggs with the milk, Parmesan cheese, olives, and nutmeg. Add the arugula. Pour the mixture into the pie shell.

Bake for 35 to 40 minutes, or until the crust is golden brown and a knife inserted in the center comes out clean.

Cut into 6 to 8 wedges and serve warm.

Paneer and Squash

SERVES 6

Paneer is a high-protein, high-calcium traditional cheese made from water buffalo's milk in India. I make paneer at home and occasionally will buy it ready-made at a natural food store. When you notice you've got a half-gallon of milk in the refrigerator that needs to be used immediately, make paneer. Serve this dish with the grain of your choice. Or eat it just as it is.

To make the paneer, you may want to begin early in the day if you plan to use it for that evening's meal. Over medium heat, bring the milk to a slow boil in a large pot. Once the milk is boiling, add the salt and lemon juice. Stir slowly with a large spoon or a whisk. Within a few minutes of adding the lemon juice, the milk should separate into curds and whey. Remove from the heat.

Place a large pot in your sink, to catch the whey. In that pot place a colander, and line it with cheesecloth. Slowly, carefully (don't burn yourself, be careful of the steam), pour the separated milk through to be strained. Lift the colander, cloth, and curds away from the pot holding the whey. Save the whey for soup stock. Leave the curds in the cloth in the colander, fold the cloth over, and place a good-sized clean stone on top of the curds, to press it. Refrigerate and allow it to press for 3 to 4 hours.

Unwrap the paneer and cut into cubes. You may use it just like tofu in any dish you please.

Continued on page 146—

PANEER
2 quarts cow's or goat's
   milk, whole or 2%

1 teaspoon sea salt

1 teaspoon fresh lemon
   juice

SQUASH DISH
1 tablespoon extra virgin
   olive oil

1/2 onion, diced

2 carrots, thinly sliced

1/2 teaspoon cumin seeds

1/4 teaspoon black mustard
   seeds

1 teaspoon ground turmeric

2 medium zucchinis, cut
   into bite-sized pieces

1 yellow squash, cut into
   bite-sized pieces

1/4 cup filtered water

1 cup chopped leafy greens,
   such as bok choy,
   mustard greens, kale,
   or Swiss chard

1 1/2 cups coconut milk

Tamari

Continued from page 145—

Heat the oil in a wok or large skillet over medium heat. Add the onion, carrots, cumin, mustard seeds, and turmeric, and sauté for 1 minute. Add the zucchini and yellow squash and water, cover, and allow to simmer for 2 to 3 minutes (remember, these varieties of squash cook quickly). Uncover and toss in the paneer, the leafy greens and the coconut milk. Replace the cover and allow to simmer for 3 to 5 more minutes, until the greens are tender, but have not lost their color—and the squash is very soft. Now season to taste with tamari. Serve hot.

Telor Bali

SERVES 6

Telor Bali is considered a main dish in Bali, where good organic eggs, from yard chickens, are very dear. Turmeric has antibacterial properties and works to heal all tissue-elements of the body. In India they say that turmeric gives the energy of the divine mother. It aids in digestion, especially of proteins. Serve this high-protein dish with rice (try Nasi Kuning, page 162) and leafy green vegetables. Also, to prepare perfect hard-boiled eggs, see page 46.

In a medium saucepan whisk the ginger, garlic, turmeric, coriander, and salt to taste into the coconut milk. Cook over medium heat for 5 to 7 minutes. When the spices have dissolved, add the eggs. Cover and simmer over low heat for 20 minutes. Serve the eggs hot with the sauce.

1 (1-inch) piece ginger root, peeled and grated

2 cloves garlic, grated

2 teaspoons ground turmeric

1/2 teaspoon ground coriander

1 teaspoon sea salt

1 cup coconut milk

6 hard-boiled eggs, peeled

2 pounds salmon fillets

1 (1-inch) piece fresh ginger, peeled and grated

6 ounces sour cream (approximately 1 cup)

2 tablespoons tamari or soy sauce

Simple Salmon Bake

SERVES 4 TO 5

You may wish to try this recipe with other kinds of fish, as well as salmon. Serve with rice, another grain, or a side of pasta. It is perfect with a salad or vegetable dish.

Preheat the oven to 350°F.

Arrange the salmon fillets in a 9-by-13-inch glass baking pan. In a small bowl, mix the ginger with the sour cream and tamari. Spread this sauce evenly over the fish fillets. Bake for about 15 to 20 minutes, or until cooked through, but not dry (baking time will depend on the thickness of fillets). Serve hot.

Salmon Burgers

SERVES 6 TO 8

This recipe comes from my mother. As a child I enjoyed the festivity of preparing and grilling salmon burgers. In Alaska, salmon is not produced on farms or genetically modified. If you cannot find fresh Alaskan salmon, use quality canned Alaskan salmon. Salmon is rich in vitamins A and B12, and in calcium, iron, magnesium, phosphorus, and potassium. Use whole-grain bread crumbs (I make my own and freeze them for later use), which are a complex carbohydrate. The eggs give this recipe a protein boost. Serve on whole-grain buns with stone-ground mustard, mayonnaise, ketchup, lettuce leaves, and tomato slices.

Preheat a grill or grill pan or set out a large cast-iron skillet.

In a large bowl, whisk the eggs. Add the salmon, bread-crumbs, and tofu, and stir to mix. Using a fork or your hands, work in the tamari, celery, and onion, and salt to taste. When the mixture is well-blended, form into 6 to 8 burger patties and dust with cornmeal. Grill the burgers for about 5 minutes on each side on the medium-hot grill or grill pan, or brown in a large cast-iron skillet with a touch of olive oil. The burgers are done when the outside is golden brown.

2 large eggs

15 ounces pink or red Alaskan salmon, baked until fork-tender (can substitute canned)

1 cup whole-grain breadcrumbs

1 cup crumbled firm tofu

3 tablespoons tamari or soy sauce

2 stalks celery, minced

1 onion, finely diced

Sea salt

¼ cup cornmeal

Olive oil (for use with skillet)

½ pound salmon, cut into
½-inch cubes

1 tablespoon olive oil

1 teaspoon tamari

1 small bunch green onions,
white and green parts,
chopped

2 cloves garlic, minced

3 tomatoes, diced

1 bunch cilantro, chopped

Juice of 1 lemon

¼ cup balsamic vinegar

Salt (to taste)

Ceviche Simple

SERVES 4 TO 6

*This high-protein salad can also be served as a main
dish on a summer day. Choose only the freshest salmon,
from a source you can trust. Because I don't recommend
raw fish for pregnant women, I cook my salmon before
marinating it.*

Braise the cubed salmon in the olive oil and tamari until
well done, but tender. In a beautiful serving bowl, toss
together all of the ingredients and allow to marinate for 2
hours or longer in the refrigerator. Serve chilled.

Mani Chicken or Tempeh

SERVES 4 TO 6

This dish is so quick and easy, it has become a standard family favorite. Now that the children are in their teen years with double the average appetite, we double the recipe. Serve with rice.

Preheat the oven to 350°F.

Place the ginger and garlic in a 9-by-13-by-2-inch glass or enamel baking dish. If using tempeh, coat the bottom of the baking dish with ¼ cup extra virgin olive oil. Arrange the chicken or tempeh on top and sprinkle with the sugar and tamari. If desired, sprinkle with pepper and paprika.

Bake for at least 1 hour, or until chicken is tender and comes off the bone easily. The tempeh will require a shorter baking time, about 40 minutes. Serve hot.

1 (2-inch) piece fresh ginger, peeled and grated

4 to 6 cloves garlic, minced

1 chicken, cut into parts, or 1½ pounds tempeh, cubed

¼ cup raw sugar or Sucanat

½ cup tamari or soy sauce

Pinch of freshly ground black pepper (optional)

Pinch of sweet paprika (optional)

2 tablespoons extra virgin olive oil

2 pounds chicken, skinned and cut into parts

2 to 4 cloves garlic, crushed

4 black peppercorns

2 bay leaves

4 to 6 white or russet potatoes, cubed

2 carrots, cut into ½-inch pieces

¾ cup apple cider vinegar

⅓ cup tamari or soy sauce

4 cups filtered water, boiling

Freshly ground black pepper

5 to 7 cups hot cooked rice

Chicken Adobo

SERVES 6

Chicken adobo is a specialty of the Philippine Islands. It is said to nourish and strengthen pregnant and breastfeeding women. It is also a dish loved by children and adults alike. This version of Chicken Adobo comes to me via my mother, who learned it from my lola. Now that I'm a lola, I've passed the recipe on to my daughter, confident that someday my granddaughter will make it for her children! If you're breastfeeding a young baby who is sensitive to the foods you eat, start with a small amount of garlic. When your baby is older, you may increase the amount.

Heat the oil in a large pot over medium heat. Add the chicken and brown the individual pieces on all sides, turning frequently to avoid burning, about 7 to 10 minutes. Add the garlic, peppercorns, and bay leaves and continue to stir. When the chicken is browned on all sides, add the potatoes, carrots, vinegar, and tamari. Allow the chicken mixture to simmer for 5 to 10 minutes. The potatoes will be about half cooked. Then add the boiling water. Let the adobo cook over medium heat until the chicken is very tender and cooked through and the potatoes are very soft, about 20 to 30 minutes. Add pepper to taste. Remove the bay leaves and serve over the rice.

Amalia's Pinakbit

SERVES 6 TO 8

Another Filipino favorite, this one-pot main dish is a unique blend of flavors that I loved in my childhood. My dear friend, Amalia, makes this simple and delicious version. Serve hot over rice, couscous, or the grain of your choice.

Place all ingredients in a large pressure cooker. Cover and place over medium heat. Shake the pot often, to blend the flavors. It takes about 30 minutes to cook through.

1 onion, cut into bite-sized pieces

2 green bell peppers, seeded and cut into bite-sized pieces

1 Japanese eggplant, cubed

½ pound green beans, trimmed and halved

1 pound tomatoes, peeled and crushed (fresh or canned)

1 bitter melon, seeded and cut into bite-sized pieces (optional)

½ pound chicken or meat of your choice, cut into bite-sized pieces (optional)

½ cup Asian fish sauce or 1 can sardines packed in olive oil

2 (2-inch) pieces fresh ginger, peeled and smashed with a pestle or hammer

Praise for Grains and Legumes

The germ is the smallest part of the grain. It is the future sprout, the seat of the grain's life potential. Without its germ and bran covering, a grain is mostly starch. With all its parts, it is a great source of complex carbohydrates, with B vitamins, vitamin E, and minerals, too.

Legumes are peas and beans, including garbanzo beans, lentils, black beans, pinto beans, soybeans, adzuki beans, black-eyed peas, mung beans, great Northern beans, kidney beans, lima beans, navy beans, peanuts, and green peas, to name a few. They are a good source of fiber, so they keep our intestines happy.

GRAINS AND LEGUMES

Grains are one of our most ancient foods. They are "fuel" for humans. Choose unrefined or whole grains, which have their bran and germ intact, so that you and your family will get the full nutritional benefit of eating grains. Pregnant and breastfeeding moms need the slow-burning, sustained sources of energy they will find in unrefined grains.

Legumes are edible plant seeds that are low in calories and high in protein. To make legumes complete proteins, meaning all the essential amino acids are present in nearly equal amounts, mix them with unrefined grains.

1 cup dried beans (pinto,
  great Northern, kidney,
  black-eyed, or garbanzo)

3 cups brown rice

Filtered water for soaking

8 cups filtered water, for
  cooking

Basic Crockpot Protein

SERVES 6 TO 8

Imagine waking up in the morning to the smell of something good cooking. Crockpots make this so easy. This recipe makes a basic protein source. When the dish has finished cooking, you can spice it up as you like, depending upon your mood. Add curry, Asian or Mexican spices, or simply serve with vegetables.

Begin in the morning, the day before you plan to eat this. Soak the beans and rice together, right in the crockpot. In the evening, before going to bed, discard the soaking water, rinse the rice and beans, replace the old water with 8 cups water or as much as will fit comfortably in your crockpot, leaving 2 inches at the top. Cook the rice and beans on the low setting all night.

About Slow-Cooking Beans

*Y*ou will need to experiment with beans. They make their own relationship with the cook. Black beans and pinto beans just seem to cooperate with Cubans, like Marina. Since I was raised by an Asian mother, mung beans and rice like me better. Pinto beans and black beans try to play with me. You'll soon get the hang of slow-cooking beans; just give it a try. It's worth the time it takes.

Adzuki Bean Gruel

SERVES 3 TO 4

6 cups filtered water

I cup adzuki beans

It is important during pregnancy (and all your life) to keep your kidneys, liver, and gallbladder functioning properly. Eating smaller meals, many times throughout the day, rather than large meals, helps balance these organs. Sugar, animal fats, overly spicey foods, margarine and hydrogenated oils, soft drinks, refined carbohydrates (like white bread), chocolate, and coffee all strain these vital organs.

This recipe has been found to help balance and cleanse the kidneys, liver, and gallbladder. It was given to me by Carole Montanari, an extraordinary doula from Long Island, New York. Her three beautiful children, Dylan, Mayan, and Suyan, are a testament to her mothering talent. Her wonderful husband Billy should be mentioned, as he makes it possible from his supportive heart for Carole to be the mother that she is. One cup a day of this gruel will encourage your organs to function better and reduce high blood pressure.

Soak the beans for 3 to 5 hours. Drain and replace the water. Bring to a boil, decrease the heat, and simmer until the adzuki beans are disintegrated, about 45 minutes to 1 hour. Put through a sieve, or blend. Serve warm or at room temperature. You may wish to sweeten the gruel with maple syrup, your favorite savory spices, or sea salt.

2 cups brown rice

I cup mung or adzuki beans

7 cups filtered water

3 to 5 fresh or dried shiitake
mushrooms

1½ tablespoons toasted
sesame oil

2 carrots, cut into bite-sized
pieces

I onion, diced (optional for
mothers with sensitive
babies)

I teaspoon ground turmeric

2 tablespoons freshly
ground black sesame
seeds

Flaxseed oil

Jeannine's Postpartum Staple

SERVES 4 TO 6

Those of you who love the book Prenatal Yoga *will feel the love in this recipe provided by Jeannine Parvati Baker. If you have not read* Prenatal Yoga *or* Conscious Conception, *please treat yourself and your family to these treasures. The flaxseed oil really makes this a wonderfully nutritious food, with those omega oils we need so much. Pregnant women in their second trimester (which is when the baby's brain is growing the fastest) would be wise to eat this.*

Rinse the rice and beans. Soak in 3 cups of the filtered water for 4 or more hours.

Meanwhile, if you are using dried shiitake mushrooms, heat the remaining 4 cups filtered water until warm. Add the mushrooms and soak them until soft, about ½ hour. Remove from the water, squeeze gently, and cut into strips. Set aside. Reserve the soaking water.

To cook the rice and beans, transfer the mixture to a large saucepan. Add the remaining 4 cups water or reserved mushroom soaking water. Bring to a boil, then lower the heat, cover, and cook until the beans are completely tender, about 1 to 1½ hours.

Heat the oil in a large cast-iron skillet to medium-high heat. Add the carrots, onion, shiitakes, turmeric, and sesame seeds, and sauté for 3 to 5 minutes, until the onions are translucent and the carrots are cooked but still firm.

In individual serving bowls mix together the rice and beans with the sautéed vegetables. Top each serving with 1 teaspoon of flaxseed oil. Serve at once.

Marina's Cuban Black Beans

SERVES 4 TO 6

Marina Alzugaray is a wonderful midwife living in Southern Florida. This recipe reflects Marina's strong ties to her culture. Black beans are suprisingly high in iron, calcium, potassium, and phosphorus. You'll also be happy to know they have thiamine, niacin, and pantothenic acid. Serve the beans over brown rice, especially with the mushrooms, and you'll have a complete protein meal. Marina says, "Make plenty, these black beans are better the next day." Serve with whole-grain tortillas for complete protein.

Drain and rinse the soaked beans, transfer to a saucepan, add the water, and bring to a boil. Transfer the mixture to a crockpot set on low heat and cook for several hours. If your beans appear dry, add boiled water. Once the beans are soft, which can take all morning, begin preparing the vegetables.

Heat the oil in a medium saucepan over medium heat. Add the onion, garlic, bell pepper, mushrooms, cilantro, and jalapeño, and sauté until the onions become translucent, about 3 minutes. Add salt to taste. Add the vegetable mixture to the cooked black beans and continue to cook in the crockpot for another 20 minutes. Serve hot.

1½ cups dried black beans, soaked overnight

3 cups filtered water

2 tablespoons extra virgin olive oil

1 onion, diced

2 to 3 cloves garlic, minced

1 green bell pepper, seeded and diced

4 ounces mushrooms, any type, thickly sliced

1 bunch fresh cilantro, chopped, stems included (optional)

1 jalapeño pepper, seeded and minced (optional)

Sea salt

1 cup dal (use chana, toovar,
   or matar—also called split
   pea dal)

1 cup quinoa

5 cups filtered water

1 teaspoon ground turmeric

Pinch of ground cinnamon

Pinch of raw sugar or
   Sucanat

Pinch of ground cardamom

Pinch of salt

½ teaspoon coriander seeds

1 teaspoon cumin seeds

1 teaspoon fennel seeds

¼ cup ghee (see page 198)

Khichari

SERVES 4 TO 6

Khichari is easy to digest and easy to make. Quinoa is a grain native to South America and rich in protein, iron, calcium, B vitamins, and other minerals. Here I've married quinoa with Indian dal to create a cross-cultural and nutritious dish.

Wash the dal and quinoa. In a large pot, bring the water to a boil. Add the dal, quinoa, turmeric, cinnamon, sugar, cardamom, and salt. Decrease the heat and simmer for about 1 hour, until the mixture has the consistency of gravy (add more water if necessary). With a mortar and pestle (or small grinder), crush the coriander, cumin, and fennel seeds. In a small saucepan, blend together ghee and crushed seeds and simmer for 1 to 2 minutes. Stir the ghee and seed mixture into the quinoa and dal. Season to taste with salt and serve.

Fried Rice

SERVES 4

This no-meat version of a traditional recipe is a favorite with my children. Mothers who wish to increase their vitamin B6 intake should make this dish with brown rice. For protein, serve fried rice with a tofu dish.

Heat the oils in a wok or large cast-iron skillet over medium-high heat. Add the garlic and ginger and sauté for 1 to 2 minutes. Decrease the heat to medium and add the carrot, onion, celery, almonds, and green beans. Sauté until the onions are translucent and the carrots become tender. Add the zucchini. When the zucchini is almost tender, add the rice, pepper, and tamari to taste. Mix well. Serve hot.

2 tablespoons extra virgin olive oil

2 tablespoons toasted sesame oil

2 cloves garlic, minced

1 (1/2- to 1-inch) piece fresh ginger, peeled and grated, or 1/2 teaspoon ground ginger

1 carrot, diced

1/2 sweet onion, diced

1 stalk celery, diced

1/2 cup slivered almonds

1/4 pound green beans, trimmed and thinly sliced

1 medium zucchini, sliced

4 cups cooked rice (brown or basmati)

Pinch of freshly ground black pepper

Tamari or soy sauce

Preparing Grains and Legumes

Wash the grains in plenty of water, swirling them in a large pot or bowl. Carefully pour off the water and repeat three times before cooking. To reduce the intestinal gas that many people experience after eating beans, soak your beans overnight, then discard the water and replace it with fresh water before cooking. This will leach out most of the fermenting properties in the coverings of the beans. Also, combining one part beans with three parts unrefined grains reduces the gas and makes your meal a complete protein.

Nasi Kuning (Yellow Rice)

SERVES 6

2 tablespoons olive oil

6 small red shallots, cut into thin rounds

¾ to 1 cup coconut milk

2 teaspoons ground turmeric

½ teaspoon ground lemongrass

½ teaspoon ground coriander

6 cups cooked basmati rice

Sea salt

1 cucumber, peeled and sliced into thin rounds

Nasi Kuning is a celebration food in Bali. It is colored with turmeric root, which is a natural antibiotic, digestive aid, and blood purifier. It is said that turmeric, when ingested, gives the energy of the Divine Mother and promotes prosperity. While promoting proper metabolism this tonic herb is good for the ligaments of the body. Is it any wonder that it's sacred? In Bali we make this dish with fresh-grated turmeric root, freshly hand-extracted coconut milk, and freshly picked lemon grass. In the United States we compromise a little, but the results are nearly as wonderful.

Heat the oil in a wok or large cast-iron skillet over medium high heat. Add the shallots and fry until they are crispy brown. Remove them from the wok and set aside on paper towels to absorb the oil.

In the same wok, combine the coconut milk, turmeric, lemon grass, and coriander. Simmer for about 15 minutes over low heat, stirring often. Add the rice, mixing as you go, so that all of it is completely yellow. Season with salt to taste.

Arrange the cucumber rounds on edge of a serving tray. Mound the rice in the center of the tray and top with the fried shallots. *Salamat hari raya!* (Blessings on your celebration day!)

Lemon Rice

SERVES 2 TO 4

Rice is soothing as it decreases the "wind" in your body. Often during pregnancy and postpartum women feel irritated or spaced-out after a day in the wind or traveling by car. (Absolutely stay off of motorbikes while pregnant or postpartum: the wind is too much, and it's not very safe.) This rice is quick to make, especially if you have some rice left over from a previous meal. The spices and lemon make it very digestible and the turmeric averts illnesses. For a light dinner, try serving Lemon Rice with Rainy Day Tomato Soup (page 124).

Heat the ghee in a large cast-iron skillet over medium heat. Add the turmeric, cumin seeds, and mustard seeds, and allow the seeds to pop without burning. Stir constantly. Add the rice and drizzle with lemon juice. Stir well and add salt to taste. Continue cooking over medium heat, stirring often, for about 5 to 7 minutes—until rice is hot. Serve hot.

2 to 3 tablespoons ghee (see page 198)

½ teaspoon ground turmeric

½ teaspoon cumin seeds

½ teaspoon black mustard seeds

3 cups cooked basmati or brown rice

2 to 3 tablespoons fresh lemon juice

Sea salt

3 tablespoons ghee (see page 198)

1 teaspoon garam masala (see page 199)

1 teaspoon black mustard seeds

$\frac{1}{2}$ cup shredded unsweetened coconut

2 to 3 cups cooked rice

1 tablespoon raw sugar, Sucanat, or raw honey

Coconut Rice

SERVES 2 TO 4

This sweet side dish pleases most palates. According to Ayurvedic medicine, coconut pacifies excess fire in the body. Excessive fire in the body causes PMS, a hot temper, and skin rashes. This rice dish is soothing and, due to the garam masala, very digestible. (Use my garam masala recipe or buy it already made at your health-food store or Asian market.) My family loves Coconut Rice with Tempeh à la Wil (page 136) and a pile of organic salad greens on the side.

Heat the ghee in a large cast-iron skillet over medium heat. Add the garam masala, mustard seeds, and coconut, and sauté until the coconut is just golden brown, about 2 minutes. Stir in the rice and sugar and cook long enough to heat through, about 5 to 7 minutes. Serve immediately.

Quinoa and Brown Rice

SERVES 6 TO 8

Quinoa is a South American grain, which is now available in North America at health-food stores. It is nutritious and well worth adding to your shopping list. At a postpartum lunch celebrating our friends Rebecca, Scott, and their new baby, Inti, I had a chance to serve quinoa. Scott's mother, Louisa, who is from Peru, wept with joy to be eating her childhood food, which she did not know existed in the Northern Hemisphere.

In a medium pot, wash the rice and quinoa three times. Add the water, cover with a snug-fitting lid, and place over high heat. Watch it carefully. As soon as it boils, decrease the heat to the lowest possible setting and allow it to simmer for 30 to 40 minutes. Follow your nose and you will begin to smell a nutty aroma; this is the grain reaching its delicious conclusion. Quickly fork out a bit, without allowing a lot of steam to escape, and taste it. If the grains are well cooked: not soggy, but just right, remove from the heat and serve.

1½ cups quinoa
1½ cups brown rice
5 cups filtered water

2 cups brown rice

½ cup kamut (available at health-food stores)

¼ cup shelled sunflower seeds

¼ cup cashews

4½ cups filtered water

Bruce's Bachelor Rice

SERVES 4 TO 6

Don't laugh—this bachelor can cook a fantastic grain. This is the best foundation for any meal. Grain cooked this way has kept its maximum amino acid, vitamin, and mineral content. Try serving it with stir-fried vegetables or mix it with beans and use it to stuff tortillas—adding tomatoes, grated cheese, salsa, and sour cream. You will need a 6- to 8-quart pressure cooker.

Soak the rice and kamut for 8 hours (or overnight) in 2½ cups water. Combine the soaked rice and kamut with the seeds and nuts in a pressure cooker with the remaining 2 cups water. Cover and turn on high heat. Listen. When the valve on top begins to rock, cook for 10 to 12 more minutes. If there is no rocker on top of the cooker, cook with medium pressure. Then turn it off. You will smell the aroma. Remove the pot from the heat, but do not open for 15 more minutes, or until you are ready to eat. Be very careful to ensure that the pressure has dissipated before opening. The grain should be well cooked, and all of the water, absorbed.

Downtown Vegetarian Chicken

SERVES 2

In Hawaii we lived on a farm, grew most of our own food, and seldom went to town. We were mostly vegetarian, except for dairy products from our own milk goats, occasional chickens (when the population of roosters got too dense), and fish. One night when our daughter Zhòu was three years old, she wanted to eat chicken. I explained that we would need to go all the way downtown (nearly a two-hour trip) to get a chicken. Instead I made this unusual oatmeal dish. She loved it and christened it "Downtown Chicken," and a family tradition was born. Oats are a complex carbohydrate, so they provide energy over a long period of time. They're also 10 to 15 percent protein and contain many vitamins and minerals. You may be surprised how nourishing and balancing this is. Try this quick dish if you wake up in the middle of the night hungry. It will boost your nutrition and allow you to get back to sleep.

2 cups filtered water

1 cup old-fashioned rolled oats

1 tablespoon nutritional yeast

Tamari

Simply cook the oats as you would prepare them for breakfast: In a medium saucepan, bring the water to a rapid boil. Use a whisk to introduce oats into the water, stirring constantly for about 2 minutes. Cover and decrease the heat to low. Let it cook until the oats are well done, about 10 to 15 minutes. Serve with the nutritional yeast and a little tamari mixed in.

4 cups finely ground spelt
flour (available in health-
food stores), whole-wheat
durum, hard red wheat, or
a blend of whole-grain
flours of your choice

Sea salt

1 large egg

Filtered water as needed

Homemade Whole-Grain Pasta

MAKES ABOUT 1½ POUNDS

Homemade pasta is not difficult to make. It is a little messy, but it's a fun project to do with the children. And they get to eat the fruit of their labor afterward. Use whole-grain flour, so that you will be eating a complex carbohydrate. Buckwheat makes fragile noodles, unless mixed with red or durum wheat. Some stores are now selling the actual whole grain, and providing a grinder (like they do for coffee beans). This gives one the opportunity to obtain truly fresh ground flour, which is so much more delicious—and healthier, too. For pasta the flour should be finely ground. Homemade pasta is delicious with any sauce, especially a sauce that has generous amounts of vegetables. Be careful not to overcook your vegetables; they should be colorful.

In a large bowl with plenty of room to play, mix the flour with a little salt (you may want to use your favorite veggie salt for this). Mound up and make a well in the center. Drop the egg into the well. Mix with your fingers until well blended. If it's too dry, add a little water. If too wet, add some more flour. Turn onto a floured board or table-top and knead for 7 to 10 minutes. It should begin to feel supple and elastic to your touch as you knead it.

Cover the dough with a kitchen towel, and let it rest for about an hour. This will make it easier to roll out. Dust with flour and roll with a rolling pin to a thickness of ⅛ to ¼ inch. If your dough is a little sticky, roll it out and let it rest until slightly dry. There is also no harm in adding flour during the rolling process, dusting it on a little at a time.

Cut the dough into strips with a pizza cutter, a zigzag cutter, or a knife. If you have a machine you can use that instead. (I found an excellent one at a garage sale.)

Cook the noodles at once or lay them on a rack to dry. Cooking the noodles at once makes the most delicious pastas. Remember homemade noodles, cooked at once, not dried, cook a lot faster (in about half the time) than the store-bought dried variety.

Cook noodles in a large pot with a generous amount of boiling water and a pinch of salt. Gently stir the pasta while you are cooking it, to prevent the noodles from sticking together. Cooking time will depend upon thickness and freshness of the pasta. The best way to determine if your pasta is done is to bite a piece. Do this quite often, until you get the feeling you want. It should be cooked through (tender), with just a trace of resistance to your teeth; this is *al dente,* as they say in Italy. Drain the pasta in a colander and serve at once, with the sauce of your choice.

1 cup wheat berries, washed

3 cups filtered water

1 tablespoon plain yogurt or
 1 teaspoon fresh lemon
 juice

Wheat Berry Wow

SERVES 2

Wheat berries make a wonderful change from rice. This dish is simple and beautiful. You can serve this hearty porridge with savory foods or sweeten it. Try it with maple syrup; it's wonderful. The yogurt or lemon juice is an agent that will partially ferment the grain; it's an ancient way of making the hearty whole grains more digestible.

In a large pot, wash the wheat berries well and drain. Add 1 cup of the water and stir in the yogurt or lemon juice. Allow the mixture to soak for 8 hours or overnight.

When you are ready to cook the wheat berries, do not drain the wheat. Bring the remaining 2 cups water to a boil in a large pot, then add the wheat berries and the liquid they soaked in. Bring back to a boil. Decrease the heat and simmer until the berries are tender, about 45 minutes. Serve hot.

BREADS

*T*here's an old saying, "As good as bread." Bread
nourishes the body and soul. In our family we serve it
warm at poetry readings and sing-along evenings.
Warm bread got us through some wicked Iowa winters.
There were days, during each of my pregnancies, when
nothing but toasted homemade bread could relieve the
nausea and balance me. I believe that every woman
becomes the God-us when she makes bread. When
you bake, your family worships you.

Basic Yeast Bread

MAKES 2 TO 3 LOAVES

- 1 tablespoon active dry yeast
- 1/3 cup raw sugar or Sucanat
- 2 tablespoons extra virgin olive oil
- 1/2 teaspoon sea salt
- 2 cups warm (105° to 115°F) filtered water
- 2 cups cooked oatmeal
- 2 cups spelt flour (available in health-food stores)
- 4 cups unbleached all-purpose flour, or 2 cups unbleached all-purpose flour and 2 cups whole-wheat or rye flour, plus additional flour for kneading

When my husband makes a big pot of oatmeal and there are leftovers, I know it's bread-baking day. This bread is nutritious and moist. Be creative and invent your own breads, using this basic recipe. A few variations follow. Legend has it that metal bowls and spoons impair the success of bread, so I avoid them. Our family seems to grow when bread is in the oven to include many friends. It is most fun to devour bread while it is still hot. Butter naturally can't be beat for a topping. We also love to mix olive oil with Parmesan cheese for dipping warm savory breads.

In a large bowl, dissolve the yeast, sugar, oil, and salt in the water. Stir in the oatmeal, then add the spelt flour, mixing well with a wooden spoon. Cover with a dish towel and let the dough rest for 30 minutes. Don't panic if you forget the time; bread making is a very forgiving process. A path to enlightenment actually.

After the first rest, mix the sponge with a wooden spoon for 108 strokes, because it is a mystical lucky number. Most recipes require 100 strokes, but like I say, "You wanna make bread, or you wanna get enlightened?" Being the queen of multitasking, I want to do both! Thus the 108 strokes. Cover again and allow the sponge to rest again for 30 to 45 minutes. It will be frothy when it has had a good nap.

Next add the 4 cups unbleached flour, one cup at a time, stirring it in with a wooden spoon. The dough will be stiff. Cover the dough with a dish towel and allow it to rise, until approximately doubled in bulk, which takes about 1 hour. The warmth or coolness of your house will determine the rising time. I like to let my bread rest and rise in a warm quiet place. (A quiet place is hard to find in my house, most days.)

Grease two baking sheets or two to three loaf pans, or dust a baking stone with cornmeal.

Once the dough has doubled in size, sprinkle ⅓ to ½ cup unbleached all-purpose or whole-wheat flour over a clean work surface. Place the dough on the flour. Put a little olive oil on your hands, and knead. Continue kneading until your arms ache; 7 to 10 minutes should be enough. The dough will become elastic. If it gets too sticky, dust it with flour and oil your hands.

Form the dough into two or three loaves, shaped as you like: rounds, oblongs, baguette style, heart shapes, and so forth. Place on the baking sheets, in the pans, or on a baking stone. Slash the tops three times for the "Mother, Maiden, and Crone" aspects of God-us to protect the bread. If you wish to make one huge braided loaf, divide the dough into three pieces and roll them into long, long snakes. Braid the snakes loosely, directly on a large baking sheet.

Cover the loaves with a dish towel and allow the dough to rise again until doubled in bulk. This can take between 30 minutes and 1 hour depending upon the environment, warmth, and other variables.

Preheat the oven to 375°F.

Bake for 40 to 50 minutes, until the loaves are golden brown and firm, and have a hollow sound when tapped on the top. Remove the loaves from the oven and turn them out onto racks to cool.

If you plan to store freshly baked bread, allow it to cool thoroughly before you wrap it in plastic.

Variety Bread Suggestions

To the facing recipe, just before adding the flour to the sponge, try any of these nutrition-boosting variations.

FRUIT & NUT BREAD

1 cup dried cranberries, raisins, or currants

1 cup walnut or pecan pieces

2 teaspoons ground cinnamon

ONION & WALNUT BREAD

1 onion, diced

1 cup walnut pieces

OLIVE & ROSEMARY BREAD

½ cup pitted kalamata olive pieces

2 tablespoons crushed fresh or dried rosemary

BASIL & GARLIC BREAD

2 generous handfuls fresh basil, finely chopped

4 cloves garlic, minced

SANTA FE BREAD

Corn kernels from 2 ears of cooked corn

Red bell pepper or any mild pepper of your choice, diced

2 cloves garlic, minced

1 cup grated Monterey Jack or cheddar cheese

1 tablespoon active dry
   yeast

1 cup warm (105° to 115°F)
   filtered water

2 cups whole-wheat or spelt
   flour (available in health-
   food stores)

1½ cups unbleached all-
   purpose flour, plus
   additional flour for
   kneading

1 teaspoon salt

2 tablespoons extra virgin
   olive oil

Cornmeal, for dusting pan or
   pizza stone

Perfect Pizza Dough

MAKES TWO 14-INCH PIZZA SHELLS

*It takes a little forethought to produce a truly wonderful
hearty homemade pizza, but it is well worth it. A few years
ago my daughter Zhòu gave me a pizza stone. What a gift!
It inspired me to be creative, and the results have been
very pleasing as well as nutritious.*

In a deep bowl, dissolve yeast in the water (this takes about
5 minutes). Using a wooden spoon, stir in the flours, salt,
and oil. Place a few drops of oil on your hands. Dust a
clean, flat surface with flour and turn out the dough onto
the surface. Knead enthusiastically for 7 to 10 minutes,
until the dough is smooth and elastic. If the dough is too
sticky to knead, dust it with flour, and re-oil your hands.

Shape the dough into a ball, place it in a large oiled
bowl, cover with a dish towel, and allow it to rise in a
warm place until doubled in size, 45 to 60 minutes.

Sprinkle cornmeal over the bottoms of two pizza pans
or pizza stones. Divide the risen dough ball in half. On a
lightly floured flat surface, roll each half into a 14-inch
circle. If you are using a cookie sheet, roll the dough out
into oblong shapes to fit your pans. Fold the dough in
half and gently tease and lift it onto the pan or the pre-
heated stone. Pinch the edges and shape so that the edges
are a little thicker; this will prevent the pizza topping
from spilling over.

The pizza dough is now ready for toppings.

Pesto Feta Pizza Topping

MAKES TWO 14-INCH PIZZAS

Prepare the pizza shells according to the recipe instructions.

Preheat the oven to 450°F. Spread the pesto sauce over pizza shells. Evenly sprinkle the feta and mozzarella cheeses on top. Sprinkle on the olives. Bake for 20 to 30 minutes. The pizza is done when the crust is golden brown; you'll have to lift it up and peek. Make sure the center of the pizza is cooked through before removing it from the oven. Allow the pizza to stand for 5 minutes before serving.

Perfect Pizza Dough (see facing page)

1½ cups New Mother Pesto (see page 206)

¾ pound feta cheese, crumbled

8 ounces mozzarella cheese, grated (2 cups)

1 cup pitted kalamata olives, halved (optional)

Perfect Pizza Dough (see
   page 174)

6 to 8 dried shiitake
   mushrooms

1½ cups hot filtered water

½ cup white or yellow miso

2 teaspoons toasted sesame
   oil

1 (1-inch) piece fresh ginger,
   peeled and grated

1 pound firm tofu, diced

½ cup finely diced scallions,
   green and white parts

Miso Pizza Topping

MAKES TWO 14-INCH PIZZAS

*This dairy-free recipe for pizza will really surprise your
family and friends. It's one of my husband's inventions,
making him the Zen master of pizza pie.*

Prepare the pizza shells according to the recipe instructions. Place the uncooked pizza shells on the pans you
intend to bake them on. Soak the mushrooms in the water
until rehydrated, 20 to 30 minutes. When the mushrooms
are soft, remove them from the water (reserving the water
for later use) and cut them into thin strips.

Preheat the oven to 450°F.

In a small, deep bowl, blend the miso and sesame oil
with ½ cup of the reserved water, using a fork or small
whisk. Add the grated ginger.

Spread the sauce over the pizza shells. Arrange the
mushroom strips and tofu evenly over the pizzas. Scatter
the scallions on top. Bake for 20 to 30 minutes.

The pizza is done when crust is golden brown; you'll
have to lift it up and peek. Make sure the pizza is cooked
through before removing it from the oven. Allow it to
stand 5 minutes before serving.

Garden Pizza Topping

MAKES TWO 14-INCH PIZZAS

I call this Garden Pizza because it's much more wonderful if you can pick the herbs, peppers, and tomatoes from your own garden plot.

Prepare the pizza shells according to the recipe instructions.

Preheat the oven to 450°F. Spread the tomato puree on top of the pizza shells. Sprinkle the herbs, onion, pepper, and tomatoes on top. Evenly sprinkle the cheeses on top. Bake for 20 to 30 minutes. The pizza is done when crust is golden brown; you'll have to lift it up and peek. Make sure the center is cooked through before removing it from the oven. Allow the pizza to stand 5 minutes before serving.

Perfect Pizza Dough (see page 174)

1 (16-ounce) can tomato puree

1 generous handful fresh basil leaves, finely chopped

½ handful fresh oregano leaves, finely chopped

1 onion, diced

1 green or red bell pepper, seeded and diced

2 tomatoes, diced

½ cup grated Parmesan or Romano cheese

8 ounces mozzarella cheese, grated

2 cups stone-ground cornmeal

½ cup barley flour

½ teaspoon cream of tartar or 1½ teaspoons natural baking powder

1 teaspoon sea salt

1 large egg

1 tablespoon extra virgin olive oil

2 cups rice milk, buttermilk, or soy milk

1 cup corn kernels

1 green or red bell pepper, seeded and diced (optional)

½ to 1 cup grated Monterey Jack or cheddar cheese (optional)

Corn Bread à la Megan

MAKES ONE 9-BY-12-INCH BAKING PAN OF BREAD

Megan, mother of Corwin, is an excellent cook and an even better friend. Enjoy this highly nutritious cornbread, which Megan makes with all-organic ingredients.

Preheat the oven to 425°F. Grease a 9-by-12-inch baking pan and dust lightly with flour.

In a large bowl, sift together the cornmeal, flour, cream of tartar, and salt. Set aside.

In a medium bowl, beat the egg, oil, and rice milk. Fold in the wet ingredients into the dry ingredients, followed by the corn and the peppers and cheese. Continue to stir mixture until well-blended. Pour the batter into the prepared baking pan. Bake for about 55 minutes, or until the edges pull away slightly from the sides of the pan and a cake tester inserted into the center comes out clean. Serve warm.

Scones

MAKES 12 TO 15 SCONES

The yogurt in these scones adds calcium, and the eggs add protein. They are nutritious and delicious, too! This recipe became popular at our house in Bali, when Ibu June Whitson was living with us and receiving babies with her wise hands in the Balinese villages surrounding Ubud. June would sing while the scones were baking. Serve the scones warm with butter or Honeyed Butter (see page 208).

Preheat the oven to 400°F. Grease two baking sheets and set aside.

In a large bowl, combine the flours with the baking powder, baking soda, and salt. Using a fork or a pastry cutter, cut in the butter until it has the texture of soft crumbs.

In a medium bowl, whisk together the eggs, yogurt, and sugar. Fold this mixture into the flour mixture and stir to combine ingredients. Add the dried fruit and nuts (or chocolate chips), stirring until evenly distributed. Do not overmix. The dough will be sticky.

Using a tablespoon, place generous spoonfuls of the dough (as uniform in size as possible) 2 inches apart on the baking sheets.

Bake for 15 to 20 minutes, until golden brown. Serve warm or transfer to wire racks to cool.

1½ cups whole-wheat flour

1½ cups unbleached all-purpose flour

2 teaspoons natural baking powder

2 teaspoons baking soda

½ teaspoon sea salt

6 tablespoons chilled butter

2 large eggs

1 cup plain or flavored yogurt, or buttermilk

2 tablespoons raw sugar or Sucanat

½ cup raisins or dried cranberries or 1 cup fresh cranberries (tart and delicious, but optional)

½ cup walnuts, chopped (optional)

½ cup chocolate chips (for celebration scones)

1¼ cups quinoa flour (available in health-food stores)

1 teaspoon sea salt

½ teaspoon natural baking powder

½ teaspoon natural baking soda

½ cup raw sugar or Sucanat

½ cup apple juice or filtered water

¼ cup ghee (see page 198) or butter

¼ cup carob powder (available in health-food stores)

¼ cup sour cream or plain yogurt

2 large eggs, separated

½ cup dried blueberries (optional)

Carob Muffins

MAKES 6 LARGE OR 12 SMALL MUFFINS

This is another fabulous recipe created by Megan. The sour cream makes these muffins very tender and mouthwatering. All-organic ingredients make this an excellent source of nutrients.

Preheat the oven to 375°F. Grease a muffin tin and dust lightly with flour.

In a large bowl, sift together the flour, salt, baking powder, baking soda, and sugar. Set aside.

Combine the apple juice and ghee in a small saucepan over medium-high heat. Bring to a boil. Remove the pan from the heat and whisk in the carob powder. Let cool slightly, then beat in the sour cream and egg yolks. In a separate bowl, beat the egg whites with an electric mixer until stiff. Stir the carob mixture into the dry ingredients. Fold in the egg whites and the blueberries. Pour the batter into the muffin tin. Bake for 25 to 35 minutes, until the muffins are lightly golden brown and a cake tester inserted into the center of a muffin comes out clean. Remove the pan from the oven and cool the muffins in the pan for 5 minutes before removing them to cool slightly on a rack. Serve warm or at room temperature.

Zucchini Cocoa Bread

MAKES ONE 8-INCH SQUARE BREAD

This simple cakelike quick bread takes only a few minutes to come together. It's perfect for a summer evening snack, when your garden is chock-full of zucchinis. The subtle flecks of green, hiding in the deep moist chocolate body of this bread, must make the God-us smile. I've been known to serve it at breakfast time. The bread also packs up nicely for a picnic. The added yogurt is high in calcium and B vitamins. It also contains protein and can aid sluggish digestion. For the almond extract, I prefer the glycerin-based, all-natural kind.

Preheat the oven to 375°F. Grease an 8-inch square (or a 9-inch round) cake pan and dust it with flour.

In a large bowl, combine the flour, sugar, cocoa powder, baking powder, baking soda, salt, and nutmeg.

In a small bowl, whisk together the eggs, zucchini, yogurt, oil, and almond extract. Fold the zucchini mixture into the flour mixture using a large wooden spoon or spatula. Do not overmix. Pour the batter into the prepared pan and arrange the pecan halves on top.

Bake for 25 to 30 minutes, until the edges pull away slightly from the sides of the pan and a cake tester inserted into the center comes out clean. Serve warm or store at room temperature, covered in plastic wrap.

1⅓ cups spelt flour (available in health-food stores)

½ cup raw sugar or Sucanat

7 tablespoons unsweetened cocoa powder

2 teaspoons natural baking powder

½ teaspoon natural baking soda

½ teaspoon sea salt

1 teaspoon freshly ground nutmeg

2 medium eggs

2 cups shredded zucchini

½ cup plain yogurt

2 tablespoons almond oil (or substitute any healthy vegetable oil)

2 teaspoons almond extract

16 pecan halves (optional)

½ cup (1 stick) butter

1 onion, diced

6 stalks celery, diced

10 ounces mushrooms,
    sliced (optional)

Tamari or seasoning salt

⅛ teaspoon freshly ground
    black pepper

1 teaspoon fresh sage,
    minced, or 1 teaspoon
    dried, crushed

½ teaspoon fresh rosemary,
    or 1 teaspoon dried,
    crushed

3 apples, cored and diced

20 ounces bread ends, diced,
    or stuffing mix

1 cup dried cranberries

½ cup diced dried papaya

1 cup macadamia nuts

Olive oil to grease baking
    dish

1 pound firm tofu, cubed
    (optional)

¾ pound cheddar cheese,
    grated (optional)

Aloha Stuffing

This stuffing came to life one Thanksgiving in Maui. Jan, my dear friend and midwife, lived in a house with two beautiful macadamia nut trees in the yard. The children discovered that they could load the nuts into the perfect-sized bubble holes of big lava rocks and hit them with a hammer. This method produced bags of shelled macadamia nuts in no time. Jan and I took to finding uses for these wonderful mac-nuts—they went into the stuffing, and a family tradition was born.

I save bread ends, cut into bite-sized pieces, in the freezer for stuffing. If you don't have a bag of bread ends in your freezer, a nice wholesome brand of dried stuffing can be found at most grocery stores. This recipe makes enough stuffing for one 15 to 20-pound bird. Or, you can make this as a vegetarian dish and bake it in a baking pan.

Preheat the oven to 350°F. Melt the butter in a large pot over medium-high heat. Add the onion, celery, mushrooms, tamari, pepper, sage, and rosemary. Sauté until the onion becomes translucent, about 3 to 4 minutes. Fold in the apples, bread cubes, cranberries, papaya, and nuts. Place the mixture into a turkey or chicken and bake in a large, greased roasting or baking dish until the fowl is well done.

To make a main-dish vegetarian stuffing, fold in the tofu. Place in a greased baking dish. Cover, and bake for about 1 hour. A few minutes before serving, uncover, sprinkle with the cheese, return the baking dish to the oven, and allow the cheese to melt. Serve hot.

SNACKS

The hour between three and four p.m. is snack-o'clock at our house. Often one or more of the mothers I received babies for will arrive with her children. I call them "my babies." Is it any wonder that one of little Chay-chay's first sentences was "Make popcorn, Robin." And so I did. Snacks, sauces, dips, spreads, and condiments do spice up our lives, and it's not difficult to make them nutritious. Enjoy!

MOLASSES POPCORN • FAIRY-GODMOTHER POPCORN • PEPITAS PARADISO
SARDINES AND CRACKERS • PUNJIRI • ANTS ON A LOG
HANOMAN'S DELIGHT • PICADILLY SILLY • SWEET POTATO CHIPS
SILKEN TOFU QUICK PROTEIN FIX • TOFU VEGGIE BALLS
AVOCADO SANDWICH

2 tablespoons extra virgin
 olive oil

I cup popping corn

Sea salt

¼ cup (½ stick) butter

½ cup blackstrap molasses

2 tablespoons cocoa powder
 (optional)

½ cup chopped almonds
 (optional)

Molasses Popcorn

MAKES 6 TO 10 SERVINGS

*This not-too-sweet treat is very high in iron and
pleasantly filling.*

Heat the oil in a large, deep (6-quart or larger) saucepan
over medium heat. Add the corn, cover, and allow to heat.
Cook, shaking the pan often, until the popping stops,
about 5 minutes. Dump the popcorn into a large bowl.
Salt to taste.

 In a small saucepan, melt the butter over low heat and
whisk in the molasses, cocoa powder, and chopped
almonds. Keep stirring with the wire whisk for 3 to 5 minutes. Drizzle the warm molasses mixture over the popcorn
while tossing and stirring the corn (you'll need some help
with this step). Serve at once.

Fairy-Godmother Popcorn

MAKES 6 TO 10 SERVINGS

Several days a week I am blessed with an afternoon visit from my godchildren, Charan and Chay-chay. When Chay-chay was born, Charan began to call me, "the Mid-life." Currently he's taken to referring to me as his "fairy god-mother." Virtually every time we get together, Chay-chay asks for popcorn. Their mom, Alesia, orders organic pop-corn from the food co-op, 25 pounds at a time, and drops it at our house. We keep our tamari in a pump spray bottle, which makes it easy to season the popcorn. Chay-chay's mommy says that this popcorn is truly magical food for the soul!

2 tablespoons extra virgin olive oil

½ cup popping corn

Tamari or soy sauce

2 tablespoons nutritional yeast

2 tablespoons beet powder (see Note)

Heat the oil in a large, deep (6-quart or larger) saucepan over medium heat. Add corn, cover and allow it to heat. Cook, shaking the pan often until the popping stops, about 5 minutes. Dump the popped kernels into a huge bowl.

Mist the popped corn with tamari to taste. Then sprinkle it with the yeast and beet powders. Mix and enjoy.

Note: Beet powder is sometimes difficult to find in stores. I order it from the local food co-op, in bulk. I get a few pounds when it is available, as beets are seasonal.

1 cup pumpkin seeds

½ cup sunflower seeds
(optional)

1 cup raisins

Tamari or soy sauce

Pepitas Paradiso

SERVES 2 TO 4

Raisins are packed with iron and pumpkin seeds are popping with life-force. This recipe presents an unusual and wonderful combination of flavors.

Heat a medium-sized cast-iron skillet over high heat. Reduce the heat to medium and add the pumpkin and sunflower seeds. Stir them often to avoid burning. When the seeds begin to pop and become slightly golden, about 2 to 4 minutes, remove the pan from the heat. Pour the seeds into a serving bowl and add the raisins. Season with tamari to taste. Serve warm or cold.

Sardines and Crackers

Did you know that the brain is mostly made of fat? This means that while you are pregnant, your baby's brain needs lipids, particularly those unsaturated fatty acids from the omega-3 family. The best way to provide your baby's developing brain with the omega-3 oil it needs to attain optimum development is to eat seafood. Sardines fall at the beginning of the seafood chain, along with pilchards, herrings, and Atlantic mackerels; therefore they are generally not polluted and safe to eat.

I ask all the pregnant women I serve as midwife to consider eating sardines. Many tell me they've never tried them. Well, most of the expectant mothers who do try sardines are quite happy to eat them.

So open a nice tin of sardines and a box of whole-grain crackers . . . settle in and snack. Your baby will be smarter for it.

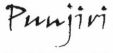

Punjiri

MAKES 1 ½ POUNDS

½ cup ghee (see page 198)

1 pound blanched almonds
(see Note)

½ pound pistachios, shelled
(optional)

1 cup dried shredded
coconut

¼ cup raw sugar or Sucanat

2 teaspoons ground
cardamom

Punjiri is traditionally given to postpartum women in India. It enhances healing and enriches breast milk. It balances and nourishes the body's tissues. This is midwife Kathy Deol's recipe. Eat 2 tablespoons each morning and evening, or snack on this whenever you're hungry.

Heat the ghee in a large cast-iron skillet over medium-high heat. Add the almonds and pistachios and roast them until they begin to turn a light golden color. Add the coconut and remove from the heat.

In a food processor or powerful blender, grind the nut mixture with sugar and cardamom. Cool before storing in a jar with a tight-fitting lid for up to 1 week.

Note: You can purchase blanched almonds, but if you wish to blanch them at home, it is easy to do: Place almonds in a pot of water, bring to a boil, drain, and let cool. Pinch each almond and the skin will slide off.

Preparing for Labor

*T*here may be no other time in your life when comfort foods are more important. Some women are ravenous during labor; others can't bear to eat a bite.

It is wise to plan ahead. My dear friend Rose made delicious loaves of cranberry-nut bread for me when I was pregnant. When she arrived to be my doula, she had two freshly baked loaves for my family and my dear midwives to eat during labor. I later found she had also stocked my freezer with cranberry-nut bread and lasagnas for my postpartum.

During labor, easy-to-digest snacks are best, as your digestion will slow down tremendously. I have found that encouraging women in labor to eat something high in calcium can take the edge off of their discomfort. Yogurt and lassi drinks made with yogurt are perfect for this. Vanilla or other flavors of soy milk, frozen into popsicles, have been a favorite treat for women who have their babies in the summer months. Try making a batch of calcium-rich red raspberry tea sweetened with honey and freezing it into ice cubes to be sucked on between contractions. This cool remedy has been known to reduce stress during labor. Red raspberry aids in the birth of the placenta, reduces the pain of afterbirth contractions, and helps new mothers produce milk.

Apricot Doula Bars (page 214) and Punjiri (facing-page) are good make-ahead snacks for you and your labor family. Ask your friends to help you out by making some healthy labor snacks and comfort foods for you.

4 to 6 stalks celery, cut into
3-inch sections

Smooth peanut butter or
almond butter

Raisins

Ants on a Log

SERVES 4 TO 6

*Sometimes it's just fun to make a snack together as a
family. When the children are small this can be frustrating.
Ants on a log is yummy and nutritious, and kids can make
it with just a little help.*

Give each child a number of prepared celery stalks on a
plate. Let them fill the concave side of each celery stalk
with the nut-butter, using a spoon. Next, let the children
line the raisins up on the nut-butter surface of the celery
stalks, just like ants on a log. This treat tastes much better
when kids make it.

Hanoman's Delight

SERVES 1

My husband, Wil, invented this extremely nutritious snack. Our son Hanoman absolutely loves it, and he's hard to please. This snack can serve as a breakfast, too.

Usually when Hanoman requests "the yogurt thing," he's so hungry that we slap the almond butter on the bread, and drizzle the honey on top of that. Top the whole thing with the yogurt and a pinch of cinnamon. This can all go into a take-away container for a picnic on those days when it's just too beautiful outside to come in and eat.

2 tablespoons almond butter or peanut butter

I slice whole-grain bread

I tablespoon raw honey or I tablespoon fruit spread (blueberry, strawberry, etc.)

¾ cup plain yogurt

Pinch of ground cinnamon

OPTIONAL GARNISHES
Raisins, dried cranberries, dried apricots (chopped), assorted nuts, bananas (sliced), peaches (cubed)

Picadilly Silly

SERVES 1

This sandwich was invented by my first grandmother-in-love, Ruth Sundt. When I heard about it, I was revolted. Once I tried it I was hooked for life. Look for a good-quality organic pickle relish at your health food store. I found that this strange combination of flavors could alleviate the worst pregnancy nausea I had. Enjoying it with a glass of milk increases the protein value.

Make it just like you would a peanut butter and jelly sandwich.

2 slices whole-grain bread (I prefer rye bread)

2 tablespoons peanut butter

2 to 3 tablespoons pickle relish

3 to 4 sweet potatoes,
    peeled and thinly sliced

Olive oil for frying

Sea salt

Sweet Potato Chips

SERVES 4 TO 6

In Indonesia it is easy to find these homemade snacks at the village warung *(little variety store). The "mother" of the store makes them early in the morning and packages them in small plastic bags. School-aged children buy them for a few* rupia *and joyfully eat them on the run. These chips are delicious served with salsa, tofu dip, or Indonesian sambal.*

Rinse the potatoes in cold water. Place them in a pot, cover with water, and bring to a boil. Decrease the heat, cover, and boil for 3 to 4 minutes. Drain the potatoes in a colander and pat them dry with paper towels.

In a skillet, heat 1 to 1½ inches of oil to fry a few sweet potato slices at a time, being careful not to allow them to smoke. Carefully, without splashing, lower a few sweet potato slices into the hot oil. Fry them, turning once or twice, until they are crisp and then drain them on paper towels (I use paper bags laid flat). Salt them to taste. Serve warm or at room temperature.

Don't Forget to Keep It Simple

When I was pregnant with Zion, who is now a handsome fifteen-year-old artist, my midwife, Jan Francisco, would always say, "Keep it simple." With three small children and one on the way, I really had to learn the Zen of cooking, cleaning, and living in general. Jan was and is a powerful teacher.

I bring this up now in the context of snacks because it's so important. When my first daughter, Déjà, was in preschool and I was in college, I learned so much from the beautiful women who worked at the school. Zoë, Clevenese, and Kathleen would say, "A child must eat a little something, every two hours." What a revelation that was to me! I've tried to make it a mothering policy around my house. Naturally when Lola (which means grandma in the Philippines, and is what my granddaughter calls me) is writing a cookbook, she needs to be reminded to feed the clan regularly. Thank heaven for Wil, a husband who loves food enough to love cooking, too.

Keeping snacks simple will mean less prep time and less clean up. You know how it is when you're busy and suddenly realize that your blood sugar is low. The children are saying, "We're hungry." And you're the only big person in sight. Yikes! The only solution is to keep it simple and make it fast.

SOME SIMPLE SNACK SOLUTIONS

Carrot sticks

Cantaloupe balls

Raisins & nuts

A banana

A banana with peanut butter

Apples—rather than apple juice, more fun to eat!

Watermelon on a hot day—eat it outside

Popcorn—eat it outside if possible

Whole-grain crackers, cheese, and strawberry slices

Just strawberries—grow them!

Just kiwifruit

A warm whole-grain tortilla with nut butter

Toast—with anything you like on it

Soy milk and wholesome cookies

A banana rolled in wheat germ—"Can I do it myself?"

Rice crackers with mashed-up avocado, topped with honey

½ teaspoon toasted sesame oil

1 (¼-inch) piece fresh ginger, peeled and grated

12 ounces soft silken tofu, cubed

1 teaspoon yellow or white miso

1 avocado, peeled and cubed (optional)

Silken Tofu Quick Protein Fix

SERVES 2

Every so often a pregnant or breastfeeding woman needs a quick protein fix. One sure sign of this need is a craving for sweets. When you crave sweets, your body often needs protein. Eating a piece of cake at a time like this will bring your energy level up temporarily, only to let you crash and burn in a matter of minutes. When my Balinese "daughter" Ketut Rusni was about to have her first baby, we discovered this quick protein fix. We found the ginger would relieve pregnancy nausea. Later in pregnancy it helped resolve heartburn.

Heat the oil in a medium saucepan over medium heat. Add the ginger and gently sauté for 1 to 2 minutes, until it begins to brown. Add the tofu and cook until just heated through, about 2 minutes. Remove the pan from the heat and stir in the miso. Garnish with the avocado, and enjoy.

Tofu Veggie Balls

MAKES ABOUT 12 BALLS

This easy-to-prepare finger food is good to take along with you when you're running errands, just in case you need an emergency protein fix. It is also rich in minerals.

Remove the tofu from the package and pat dry. In a large bowl, mash the tofu with your hands. Add the almond butter, carrots, ginger, nori, yeast, and tamari, and mix well. Form 1-inch balls in the palms of your hands. If the mixture is too wet to work with, add more nutritional yeast. Eat immediately or store in an airtight container in the refrigerator for up to 3 days.

1 pound firm tofu

¼ cup almond butter

3 carrots, finely grated

1 (½-inch) piece fresh ginger, peeled and finely grated

2 sheets toasted nori seaweed, cut into tiny strips

2 tablespoons nutritional yeast (flakes or powder), or more as needed

½ teaspoon tamari or soy sauce

1 ripe avocado

Sea salt

Squeeze of lemon

2 slices whole-grain bread

2 slices ripe tomato

2 to 3 lettuce leaves

1 handful of sprouts

2 slices of Jack or cheddar
cheese (optional)

Avocado Sandwich

SERVES 1

Often I see nursing mothers who are just plain too thin. This happens when the baby is getting bigger, around 9 to 12 months old, and is not really eating much food yet. The emerging toddler needs a lot of calories, now that she is crawling and taking steps. These additional calories are extracted from Mother, via her milk. I urge these mothers to eat avocados. One avocado contains about 300 calories, and 4 to 5 grams of protein. Avocados provide B vitamins, folic acid, and niacin, along with vitamins C, A, and E.

Open the avocado, remove the seed, and scoop the flesh out into a small bowl. Add salt to taste and a squeeze of lemon juice. Mash with a fork until well-blended but still lumpy.

Spread the avocado mixture on both slices of bread. It's moist, so you don't need mayonnaise. Layer tomato, lettuce, sprouts, and cheese over the avocado and enjoy.

DIPS, SPREADS, AND CONDIMENTS

By simply preparing an interesting dip, spread, or condiment, you can add flavor sensations from around the world to any occassion. I invite you to sample tastes of Indonesia, the Middle East, and Mexico right in your own kitchen. Try serving these recipes on crackers, bread, pasta, or even pancakes—each one is guaranteed to jazz up your next eating adventure.

GHEE • SESAME GOMASHIO • GARAM MASALA • INDONESIAN SAMBAL
DÉJÀ'S MANGO SALSA • DÉJÀ'S STANDARD RED SALSA
MIDDLE EASTERN MINT CHUTNEY • CAREE'S CRANBERRY RELISH
GARLIC SPREAD • SUN-DRIED TOMATO PESTO • NEW MOTHER PESTO
ROASTED RED PEPPER PASTE • HONEYED BUTTER
BECCA'S CARROT BUTTER • ISKANDAR'S ASPARAGUS SPREAD
FRIDAY MORNING TOFU DIP • MACADAMIA NUT DIP

Ghee

MAKES 2 CUPS

Ghee, also called clarified butter, is easy to make and can be stored in the refrigerator for a long time. Therefore you may wish to make it in large batches so you have it on hand when you wish to cook with it. It enhances "ojas" in the body. As I understand it, "ojas" is the glue of the universe. It is the love that holds all life together. It is the Ayurvedic term for oxytocin, a hormone that is richly passed from mother to baby in the last month of pregnancy. It's generally good stuff.

1 pound (or more) butter

Heat a medium saucepan over low heat. Add the butter and allow it to melt for about 15 minutes. It should have a golden color and a nice aroma. Slowly pour this liquid, and the foam on top, into a jar for storage, discarding the sediment at the bottom of the pan. Viola, you have ghee!

Sesame Gomashio

MAKES 1 CUP

Sesame seeds are rich in calcium, something every woman needs.

1 cup white or light sesame seeds

½ teaspoon sea salt

Place the sesame seeds in a skillet over medium-high heat. Toss them continuously in the skillet until they begin to turn a light golden color, about 2 to 3 minutes. Add the salt. Grind the mixture in a grinder or with a mortar and pestle. Let cool. Store in an attractive jar, right on your table, so you use it generously to flavor your food.

Garam Masala

MAKES ABOUT ½ CUP

Garam masala is the traditional Indian name for mixed spices, which can be used to flavor teas, chutneys, and savory or sweet recipes. This particular mix of spices is my favorite. You may wish to experiment with your own garam masala combination. During pregnancy and post-partum, the wind in the body can become irritated easily; cooking with garam masala spices can pacify many pregnancy discomforts by alleviating wind irritation in the body. These spices also aid digestion, helping relieve the heartburn of late pregnancy. Use the highest-quality fresh spices that are not irradiated. I buy the whole spices and grind them myself in a small spice mill.

Mix all ingredients together. Store at room temperature in a jar with an airtight lid.

2 tablespoons ground cinnamon

I tablespoon ground ginger

I tablespoon ground cardamom

I tablespoon ground coriander seed

I tablespoon ground nutmeg

¼ teaspoon ground cloves

2 tablespoons extra virgin
olive oil

2 hot green chiles (I use
jalapeño peppers), seeded
and diced

1 hot red pepper, such as
habanero, seeded and
diced

4 cloves garlic, diced

4 small shallots, diced

2 large tomatoes, diced

1 tablespoon shrimp paste
(available in Asian
markets), or 2
tablespoons Asian
fish sauce (available in
Asian markets)

1 tablespoon palm sugar
(available in Asian or
Mexican markets) or
brown sugar

1/2 teaspoon sea salt

Indonesian Sambal

MAKES ABOUT 1½ TO 2 CUPS

This is a standard condiment in Indonesian cuisine. In hard times, a poor meal can always be spiced up with a good sambal. Sambal is Indonesia's salsa. Warning: It is hot!

Heat 1 tablespoon of the oil in a wok over medium-high heat. Add the chiles, garlic, and shallots and sauté for 5 minutes until soft. Transfer this to a mortar and set aside.

In the same wok (no need to wash it between steps), using the remaining tablespoon of oil, sauté the tomatoes and shrimp paste for about 5 to 7 minutes, until the tomatoes are quite soft. Add this to the mortar containing the chile mixture.

When the mixtures waiting in the mortar are cool enough to work with, top with the sugar and salt, and grind with a pestle until smooth. *Enak sekali.* (Delicious really.) Store in an airtight container in the refrigerator. Serve at room temperature.

Dèjà's Mango Salsa

MAKES ABOUT 6 CUPS OF SALSA

This is my daughter's masterpiece. It turns any burrito, enchilada, taco, or tostada into a gourmet meal. It makes a great appetizer with tortilla chips or quesadillas. It can also dress up any main dish—try it with grilled fish or chicken. It's packed with vitamins and minerals, a living food that makes you want to dance.

In a medium bowl, toss all the ingredients together. Chill and serve.

2 large mangos, peeled, pitted, and cubed

½ red onion, finely diced

2 avocados, peeled and cubed

4 tomatoes, diced

½ cucumber, peeled and diced

1 to 2 fresh jalapeño peppers, seeded and minced

¼ cup fresh cilantro, stemmed and chopped

Juice of 2 lemons

¼ teaspoon ground cumin

½ teaspoon sea salt

6 medium tomatoes, cubed

½ onion, diced

I bunch cilantro, stemmed
and chopped

I to 2 fresh jalapeño
peppers, seeded and diced

Juice of 2 limes

½ teaspoon sea salt

Dēja's Standard Red Salsa

MAKES ABOUT 4 TO 5 CUPS OF SALSA

South-of-the-border food can brighten any gloomy day, or make a sunny summer day even warmer. Because this salsa is so full of nutrients, it's not just for fun.

Place all of the ingredients in a blender and pulse to chop. You don't want to puree this salsa, just chop and mix. Chill unless you can't wait to eat it!

2 cups tightly packed fresh
mint leaves

¼ cup fresh lemon juice

¼ cup extra virgin olive oil

4 cloves garlic

Pinch of sea salt

Middle Eastern Mint Chutney

MAKES 1 ½ CUPS

This fresh mint chutney makes a lovely relish with any meal. My family also likes it on crackers or with bread sticks. It is a traditional relish in Lebanese cuisine. Try it with Lebanese Potato Salad (page 89).

Combine the mint, lemon juice, oil, garlic, and salt in a food processor. Process until blended. Serve at once or store in an airtight container in the refrigerator for up to 4 days.

Caree's Cranberry Relish

SERVES 4 TO 6

Traveling with Ibu Caree to Bali was a true treat. She's one of my favorite poets and a sister to me. The highlight was waking her up at midnight to help me catch a baby for Ketut Kamarini. We all bonded over the birth. Caree shares a vitamin C-rich side dish, which will aid digestion. I also found this relish to be a good nausea buster and appetite stimulant in the first trimester. This makes a lumpy sweet and tart cranberry relish. Serve warm as an accompaniment with an entrée or try spreading it on toast.

In a medium saucepan, combine the cranberries, apples, pecans, cinnamon, nutmeg, salt, and grape syrup. Bring the mixture to a boil, then cover, reduce to a simmer, and cook until the apples and cranberries are tender and the flavors have blended, about 15 minutes. Remove the cinnamon stick before serving.

10 to 12 ounces frozen or fresh cranberries

2 apples, peeled, cored, and diced

1 cup chopped pecans

1 stick cinnamon

1/4 teaspoon freshly grated nutmeg

Pinch of sea salt

1/2 cup grape syrup or concentrated grape juice

I head fresh garlic

1½ cups extra virgin olive oil

½ cup grated Parmesan cheese

Garlic Spread

MAKES ABOUT 2 CUPS OF SPREAD

My family first tried this recipe at the Bread and Puppet Resurrection Circus, in Vermont. It has become an old standby at our house, where on any given night mothers, babies, fathers, poets, musicians, and roustabouts may show up hungry. Any bread becomes a feast when served with garlic spread and tea.

Separate the garlic into individual cloves and peel. Mince the garlic as finely as possible. Place the garlic in a medium mixing bowl, and add the olive oil and Parmesan cheese. Mix well and serve in two shallow bowls.

Sun-Dried Tomato Pesto

MAKES ABOUT 4 CUPS

This is a wonderful recipe to serve when entertaining people who prefer to eat mostly raw foods. The tomatoes, which contain potassium, vitamins C, E, and A, folic acid, biotin, niacin, and minerals, are dried by the power of the sun, not cooked on a stove.

Soak the sun-dried tomatoes in the water for 1 to 4 hours. Drain, reserving the soaking water. Combine the soaked tomatoes, walnuts, garlic, oil, cheese, and salt to taste in a food processor. Begin to process, adding the soaking water a little at a time, to achieve the desired consistency. A thick paste is wonderful as a spread for crackers or French bread. A thin paste works well for serving with pasta. Store in an airtight container in the refrigerator for up to 4 days.

¾ cup sun-dried tomatoes

3 cups filtered water

½ cup walnuts

3 to 4 cloves garlic

½ cup extra virgin olive oil

¼ cup freshly grated Parmesan cheese (optional)

Sea salt

¾ cup extra virgin olive oil

3 to 4 cloves garlic

2½ to 3 cups firmly packed basil leaves

½ cup pine nuts, walnuts, or cashews

½ cup grated Parmesan cheese

Juice of ½ large lemon

Sea salt or tamari

New Mother Pesto

MAKES 2½ TO 3 CUPS

Basil is called tulsi *in India, where it is a sacred, highly regarded healer from the plant kingdom. Basil improves elimination; strengthens the nervous system; reduces fever; hastens healing; relieves spasms; dispels colds, coughs, congestion, and headaches; and tastes wonderful! This herb is said to be life-giving. It opens the heart and mind while increasing love and devotion. (Feed this dish to your husband!)*

The cheese and nuts provide protein and calcium along with many other nutrients. Garlic is a powerful detoxifier and rejuvenator.

Serve over hot pasta as a main dish, with a side of fresh vegetables or salad. Refrigerate leftover pesto; spread on toast and eat it as a snack. For a quick high-energy lunch, use pesto as a topping over brown rice or any other whole grain.

Heat 1 tablespoon of the oil in a small saucepan or skillet over medium-high heat. Add the garlic and stir continuously until golden brown, about 1 to 1½ minutes.

In a blender or food processor, combine the remaining olive oil and basil and process until finely chopped. Gradually add the nuts, cheese, sautéed garlic, lemon juice, and salt to taste. Blend until smooth. Use immediately, or store in an airtight container in the refrigerator for up to 3 days.

Roasted Red Pepper Paste

MAKES 1½ CUPS

In Bali we have beautiful long thin red peppers, called lombok, which are not too hot. While in the United States, I've obtained organic Big Bertha or mild Italian red peppers from the garden of my dear friend Diana. This pepper paste is wonderful on toast, or try it as a dip for raw veggies.

½ pound mild red peppers
4 cloves garlic
¼ cup extra virgin olive oil
Sea salt

Roast the red peppers over a barbecue grill or on a gas stove with the flame set at medium-high. I use a small rack that fits over my gas burner to roast peppers, or I roast them individually by sticking one on the end of a fork and turning over the flame until all parts of the pepper are thoroughly charred. Remove the peppers from the flame and soak them in cold water to allow them to cool. Under cold running water, rub the charred skin off and discard. Open the peppers and remove the stem and seeds. Next, roast the garlic cloves in their peels, by piercing them with a fork and holding close to a flame for about 1½ minutes.

Place the roasted pepper in the blender. Peel the roasted garlic and place into blender with the oil and salt to taste. Blend the mixture until smooth. Serve at once or store in an airtight container in the refrigerator for up to 4 days.

½ cup (1 stick) butter, softened

3 to 4 tablespoons raw honey

2 teaspoons natural almond extract

¼ teaspoon ground cinnamon

Honeyed Butter

This sweet butter is delicious on scones, muffins, or any warm bread.

In a medium mixing bowl, combine the butter, honey, and almond extract with a fork, mixing until smooth. Transfer to a serving bowl, dust with the cinnamon, and serve.

5 medium carrots, sliced

½ cup sesame tahini

1 teaspoon arrowroot powder

1 teaspoon ground cinnamon

½ teaspoon sea salt

Becca's Carrot Butter

MAKES ABOUT 2 CUPS

This slightly sweet spread is made with sesame tahini, which makes it rich in calcium, protein, vitamins A and E, zinc, copper, magnesium, phosphorus, iron, and potassium. In the Middle East, sesame seeds are called the "seed of immortality." Try this spread on muffins, crackers, freshly baked bread, pancakes . . . imagine the possibilities.

Bring a pot of water to a boil. Add the carrots, cover, and boil them until they are tender, about 7 to 9 minutes. Drain. In a blender or food processor, combine the carrots, tahini, arrowroot, cinnamon, and salt and process until creamy and smooth. Enjoy.

Iskandar's Asparagus Spread

MAKES ABOUT 2 CUPS

After I received a baby for our friend Ade, her brother, Iskandar, an organic farmer in upland Bali, began delivering several kilos of fresh asparagus to our house every week. This abundance of asparagus caused me to begin experimenting with it. Well, I have been told this spread is food nirvana!

In a blender or food processor, combine the asparagus, scallions, ¼ cup oil, and salt to taste and process until creamy and smooth. If you use a blender, it will take more time, as you will need to turn it off, stir up the contents and then continue to blend. If it's too dry, add more olive oil, a little at a time, until it becomes smooth. Asparagus spread may be stored in the refrigerator for up to 4 days and can be eaten as a spread or as a topping for any vegetable or grain dish.

I pound fresh asparagus, tough ends trimmed and steamed, then sliced into I-inch pieces

3 to 4 scallions, diced

¼ to ⅓ cup extra virgin olive oil

Sea salt

1 pound firm tofu, cut up
   into eighths

3 cloves garlic, chopped

1 handful fresh parsley,
   chopped

1 green bell pepper, seeded
   and chopped

1 tablespoon extra virgin
   olive oil

1/2 teaspoon dried or fresh
   tarragon

1/2 teaspoon dried or fresh
   dill

1/2 teaspoon sea salt

Friday Morning Tofu Dip

MAKES 2 1/2 CUPS

I call this "Friday Morning Tofu Dip" because I know that by Friday evening my house will fill up with teen-agers. (Four of our children are now between the ages of 14 and 17, the magic of a blended family!) I don't mind that our house is the hang-out, and believe me, we go through a lot of snacks. Friday morning is a great time to throw together a nutritious snack that the children will enjoy later. Try this dip with corn chips or as a spread on your favorite toasted whole-grain bread.

In a food processor or powerful blender, combine all of the ingredients and blend until smooth. Store in an airtight container in the refrigerator for up to 3 days.

Macadamia Nut Dip

MAKES ABOUT 3 CUPS

Kathy Warner and her beautiful daughter Tiera were on hand one winter morning to celebrate the birth of our friend Mary's new son. Being a raw food chef and healer, naturally Kathy brought the food. This amazing sprouted macadamia nut dip was the perfect quick-fix energy food. Nuts are a good source of protein, rich in minerals as well. This dip requires a little planning ahead, as the nuts must be soaked and sprouted for 12 hours. However, the preparation time is only a few minutes. It keeps for days in the refrigerator, but don't count on having leftovers—once it's served, it's such a favorite. Serve with homemade bread or vegetables.

Soak the macadamia nuts in water for 12 hours. This essentially sprouts them. Rinse well. Store in an airtight container in the refrigerator for up to 4 days.

Combine the dates, tamari, coriander, caraway, lemon juice, vinegar, curry powder, and dill in a food processor or blender. Process, adding the nuts ½ cup at a time and water as needed to create a desirable consistency. I prefer this dip to be a little more liquidy than your typical nut butter, for easy dipping.

2 cups raw shelled macadamia nuts

2 cups filtered water

2 to 3 pitted Medjool dates

2 tablespoons tamari

1 tablespoon coriander seeds

1 teaspoon caraway seeds

1 teaspoon fresh lemon juice

½ teaspoon apple cider vinegar (optional)

1 teaspoon curry powder (optional)

Sprigs fresh dillweed (optional)

Sweets Sweeten the Person

Ayurvedic medicine tells us that sweets sweeten the person. Once, when my first two children were nine and five years old, I had an awakening regarding desserts. Déjà, my eldest, called a dear friend who was a therapist. She asked Joan for an appointment for family therapy. I was surprised when Joan informed me that we were meeting together with her for a family-therapy session. That Sunday, as Déjà, my son Noël, and I sat in a circle with Joan, I heard their one and only complaint about me as a mother: I was not providing them with any desserts.

I had to admit that as a single mom (which I was at that time), I was not thinking much about sweets. I had little or no craving for them and had forgotten that children, and indeed many people, really enjoy a treat now and again. We happily negotiated and came to an agreement that as a family we would make healthy desserts a part of our food repertoire.

I soon found out that the Ayurvedic theory that sweets sweeten the person was indeed true about myself. I felt more cheerful after including something sweet in my diet now and again.

WISE WOMAN DESSERTS

*P*erhaps these desserts will cheer you up and sweeten
your family, too. When lovingly prepared with
wholesome ingredients, desserts are not junk food.
In fact, most of the desserts in this chapter are
so nutritious that they're just plain good for you.

APRICOT DOULA BARS • NOËL'S DESIRE . . . CHOCOLATE CHIP COOKIES
AUNT GETTY'S GINGER SNAPS • GINGER CHOCOLATE COOKIES
WIL'S WILD BERRY CRUMBLE • AVOCADO CHOCOLATE PIE
LONI & MICHAEL'S INCREDIBLE CHOCOLATE TOFU PIE
BALI BUDDHA RAW TROPICAL PIE • PIE CRUST • APPLE PIE
TRADITIONAL PUMPKIN PIE • CHAY-CHAY'S CARROT CAKE
BAKED APPLES À LA SOPHIA • SURREAL'S DELIGHT • MAUI GINGER BREAD
JUDY'S CHOCOLATE CHIP BANANA BREAD • MANGO ICE CREAM
BASIL ICE MILK • TONI'S DATE BALLS

1/4 cup (1/2 stick) butter, at room temperature

1 tablespoon raw sugar or Sucanat

1/2 teaspoon sea salt

1/2 cup apple juice concentrate

1 1/2 teaspoons natural vanilla extract

1 1/2 cup spelt flour (available in health-food stores)

1 cup flaxseed meal (whole flaxseeds may be ground at home in blender)

1/2 pound dried figs

1/2 pound dried apricots

1/2 cup filtered water

2 tablespoons ground almonds (whole almonds may be ground in blender or small grinder)

Apricot Doula Bars

SERVES 10 TO 12

This nutritious treat was created by my friend Megan Robinson. She was wise enough to make up these "energy bars" a few days before going into labor with her son, Corwin. Megan and the birth team really enjoyed the sustenance, which is why I call them Apricot Doula Bars. Like a doula, this dessert really mothers the mother. This recipe will come in handy for moms who are simultaneously breast-feeding a wee one and juggling bigger children. Imagine how handy these will be at a soccer game. Thank you, Megan!

Preheat the oven to 350°F. Butter a baking sheet.

In a medium bowl, cream the butter with the sugar, salt, apple juice concentrate, and vanilla extract. Add the spelt flour and flaxmeal and mix well. Form the dough into two rectangular log shapes. Wrap each log in waxed paper and chill for 1 hour.

Combine the dried figs and apricots in a medium saucepan and cover them with the water. Bring the mixture to a boil, decrease the heat to a simmer, and cook until the fruits are soft, about 10 to 15 minutes covered. Remove the pan from the heat and puree the mixture with a fork. Add the ground almonds and stir to blend.

Remove the dough from the refrigerator and roll out one dough log out on the prepared baking sheet. Spread the pureed fruit and nut mixture over the dough. Roll out the second dough log onto waxed paper, cut to approximately the size of a baking sheet (10" by 14½"). Place this layer on top of the baking sheet with the dough and fruit mixture. Press lightly. Trim the edges as needed.

Bake for 15 to 30 minutes, until the bars are golden brown on top. Cut them into squares while they're still hot.

Noël's Desire... Chocolate Chip Cookies

MAKES ABOUT 4 DOZEN COOKIES

A classic favorite around our house, baked with love.

Preheat the oven to 375°F. Lightly grease two cookie sheets.

In a large bowl, cream together the butter and sugar until smooth. Beat in the eggs and the almond and vanilla extracts.

In another bowl, mix together the flour, baking powder, and salt until well-mixed. Stir in the oats. Combine the dry ingredients with the wet ingredients and blend together with a wooden spoon or spatula. Stir in the chocolate chips, white chocolate chunks, and walnuts. Drop by the spoonful onto the prepared cookie sheets, about 1½ inches apart.

Bake for 12 to 15 minutes, until edges are golden. Remove from the oven and let cool for 1 minute. Use a metal spatula to slide each cookie off the baking sheets and lift onto a cooling rack. Yum.

- I cup (2 sticks) butter, at room temperature
- I½ cups raw sugar or Sucanat
- 4 large eggs
- 2 teaspoons natural almond extract
- I teaspoon natural vanilla extract
- 3 cups whole-wheat flour
- 2 teaspoons natural baking powder
- 2 teaspoons sea salt
- 2 cups quick-cooking oats
- 8 ounces semi-sweet chocolate chips
- 6 ounces white chocolate chunks
- I cup walnuts, coarsely chopped

¾ cup (1½ stick) butter

¼ cup blackstrap molasses

1 cup raw sugar or Sucanat, plus additional for coating the cookies

1 large egg

2 cups whole wheat or spelt flour

2 teaspoons baking soda

1 teaspoon ground cinnamon

½ teaspoon ground cloves

½ teaspoon ground ginger

½ teaspoon sea salt

Aunt Getty's Ginger Snaps

MAKES ABOUT 2 DOZEN COOKIES

My dear friend Mary Kroeger is an international mid-wife, working these days mostly in Africa, Central America, and Cambodia to help slow the spread of HIV/AIDS. Her mother was from the South. Georgia, to be exact. One of Mary's favorite cookie recipes came from her Aunt Getty, Mary's mother's paternal auntie. Getty wore long pants years before it was acceptable for Southern women to do so, and Mary's mother remembers seeing her brandish her shotgun and shoot a rattlesnake that had crept into the house. The recipe uses blackstrap molasses, which is a good source of iron and calcium.

Preheat the oven to 350°F. Grease two baking sheets.

Melt the butter in a 4-quart saucepan over low heat. Remove from the heat and allow to cool. Add the molasses, sugar, and egg. Beat well.

In a medium bowl, sift together the flour, baking soda, cinnamon, cloves, ginger, and salt. Add to wet mixture and stir well.

Chill until firm.

Form into one-inch balls and roll in sugar. Place the cookies on the prepared baking sheets about 2 inches apart.

Bake for 8 to 10 minutes until edges appear dry. Use a metal spatula to lift the cookies from the pan onto a cooling rack. Enjoy.

Ginger Chocolate Cookies

MAKES ABOUT 2 DOZEN COOKIES

These cookies are good nausea busters, and they're not too sweet. The molasses contains iron, the ginger aids digestion, and the chocolate satisfies that craving.

Preheat the oven to 350°F. Grease two baking sheets and set aside.

In a medium bowl, cream the butter with the molasses, sugar, and eggs. Stir in the ginger.

In a separate bowl, sift together the flour, oats, baking soda, salt, and nutmeg. Add the dry ingredients to the wet, then add the chocolate chips and nuts. Drop spoonfuls of the batter onto the prepared baking sheet about 1½ inches apart. Bake for 12 to 14 minutes. Cookies are perfectly done when chewy, but not hard (after cooling). Lift cookies off baking sheet with metal spatula and cool on racks.

¾ cup (1½ sticks) butter, at room temperature

⅓ cup blackstrap molasses

½ cup raw sugar or Sucanat

2 large eggs

1 (1-inch) piece fresh ginger, peeled and grated

2 cups whole wheat or spelt flour

½ cup quick-cooking oats

2 teaspoons baking soda

½ teaspoon sea salt

1 teaspoon ground nutmeg

¾ cup chocolate chips

½ cup coarsely chopped pecans (can substitute walnuts or cashews)

A Note from Mary

*H*ere's another "sweet tooth" recipe I give pregnant women who are craving ice cream (which *many* of my mothers do). Instead of indulging in ice cream, I suggest plain yogurt (either low or full-fat) with a generous amount of molasses and a few raisins added. This seems to cover the ice-cream urge, and it's a healthy source of calcium, iron, and lactobacillus, which aids digestion.

FILLING

1 (2-inch) piece fresh ginger, peeled and grated

2 tablespoons fresh lemon juice

15 apples or pears, peeled, cored, and sliced (if you use small apples you will need more of them)

2 pints mulberries, raspberries, or cranberries (any fresh or frozen berries will do, and you may mix them)

¼ cup unbleached all-purpose flour

¼ to ½ cup raw sugar or Sucanat

2 teaspoons natural almond extract

CRUMBLE TOPPING

1½ cups unbleached flour

¾ cup raw sugar or Sucanat

1 teaspoon ground nutmeg

1 teaspoon ground cinnamon

½ teaspoon salt

½ cup (1 stick) butter, chilled

2 cups coarsely chopped mixed nuts (try walnuts, pecans, filberts, almonds, or pumpkin seeds)

Wil's Wild Berry Crumble

SERVES A CROWD OF 16

My husband has made himself quite popular with this recipe. When the midwives or La Leche League meet, they ask me to beg him to make us a wild berry crumble. We have one of those gadgets that peels, cores, and slices apples, and the children love to do that part of the job. Wil bakes the crumble in a huge shallow stoneware bowl, but a 15-by-10-inch baking pan will also work. When we are in the United States we core, peel, slice, and freeze apples and pears in the fall. Later, when winter mornings prevent anyone from leaving the house, Wil graces us with the aromatherapy of his berry crumble cooking. Eating it is only half the fun. Serve with a scoop of plain yogurt for the additional calcium.

Preheat the oven to 375°F.

In a small bowl, combine the ginger and lemon juice to make a sauce. Set aside. In a large pan (do it right in the dish you plan to bake in), mix the fruit with the flour, sugar, and almond extract. Pour the ginger-lemon sauce evenly over it and toss a little.

To make the crumble topping, combine the flour, sugar, nutmeg, cinnamon, and salt in a medium bowl. Cut in the butter, using two butter knives, until crumbly. This will take a little practice, but it's fun. Add the nuts and mix.

Sprinkle the crumble mixture over the fruit in the baking dish. Position the dish in a rack in the center of the oven and bake until you can see juices bubbling from a golden brown top, 60 to 70 minutes. Serve warm.

Avocado Chocolate Pie

SERVES 6

When Marina was expecting a new baby, she sent me the recipe for this wonderful dessert. She says, "I found it via the 'hungry mama' grapevine, so I won't take credit for it. I heard it came to the originator in a dream."

To make the pie crust, combine the nuts and dates with the spices in a blender or food processor and process until a sticky mixture is formed. If you are using a blender, this takes patience, and you will need to stop your blender a few times to stir up the mixture. Press the mixture into a 9-inch pie plate.

To make the filling, combine the avocado, cocoa powder, sugar, and vanilla in a blender or food processor and process until all the lumps are gone. You should have a smooth, pudding-like texture.

Spoon the filling into the prepared crust. Top with sliced fruits, dust with cardamom powder, and garnish with a sprig of mint. You may also top with some chopped nuts.

CRUST

1½ cups raw nuts, such as almonds, walnuts, pecans, or cashews

5 to 7 dates

Pinch of ground cinnamon

Pinch of ground nutmeg

FILLING

3 ripe but firm avocados, peeled and chopped

¼ cup cocoa powder

3 tablespoons raw sugar or Sucanat

1 teaspoon natural vanilla extract or natural almond extract

Fruit slices (berries, mangoes, kiwi fruit, or bananas), for topping

Ground cardamom, for dusting

Sprig of mint, for garnish

Chopped nuts, for garnish (optional)

CRUST

1½ cups pecans

6 to 8 pitted dates

Pinch of ground cinnamon

Pinch of ground nutmeg

FILLING

1 to 1¼ pounds soft tofu
(or 1 pound firm tofu plus
6 to 8 tablespoons)

1 cup chocolate chips

2 teaspoons almond extract

¼ cup raw sugar or Sucanat

OPTIONAL TOPPINGS

Strawberries, sliced

Bananas, sliced

Mangoes, cubed

Kiwifruit, sliced

¾ cup plain yogurt mixed
with 2 tablespoons honey

Edible flowers, for garnish

Loni & Michael's Incredible Chocolate Tofu Pie

MAKES ONE 9-INCH PIE

I first met Loni when she was 18 months old. Her mother, Leslie, and I were dear friends. Years later, what a joy it was one fine night to receive Loni's first baby, Lily. It makes me cry to remember Leslie's tears as she became a grandmother. This recipe is a family favorite from Loni and her husband, Michael.

To make the crust, combine the nuts, dates, cinnamon, and nutmeg in a blender or food processor and process until a sticky, crunchy mixture is formed. This takes patience; you will need to stop and start your blender many times and stir in between. Press the mixture into a 9-inch pie plate.

To make the filling, combine the tofu, chocolate chips, almond extract, and sugar in a medium bowl, and mix with a spoon until the ingredients are integrated. Spoon the filling into the pie plate and top with any or all of the fruit and yogurt. Garnish with edible flowers.

Alternate Fillings

Combine 3 cups firm tofu, 8 to 10 tablespoons soy milk, ¼ cup pure maple syrup, 6 to 7 tablespoons cocoa powder, and 2 teaspoons almond extract. Or combine 3 cups firm tofu, 6 to 8 tablespoons pineapple juice, ¼ cup pure maple syrup, and ½ cup crushed pineapple. Top with crushed pineapple, and any combination of tropical fruit such as shredded coconut, sliced bananas, fresh mango, papaya, or kiwifruit.

Alternate Crusts

Combine 1½ cup walnuts and 6 to 9 dried apricots (depending upon size and dryness). Or combine 1 cup cashews, ½ cup dried shredded coconut, and 5 to 11 pieces of assorted dried fruit, such as dates, dried papaya, raisins, figs, or prunes.

Our village in Bali is dotted with tiny stores called *warungs*. Modern times have brought packaged candies, made with refined sugar, to our *warungs*. These *manisan* (sweets) sell for a few *rupiah*. As a result, the teeth of the village children are rotting. The *warungs* are gathering places, and naturally my children find themselves there with their friends and a few *rupiah* in their sweaty hands.

The *Ibu* (mother) who runs the *warung* also sells her homemade sweets, small rice cakes made with freshly grated coconut and dark palm sugar, bags of frozen tamarind-sweetened mung beans, and boiled bananas served on a banana leaf.

Fortunately it has not been difficult to convince my children to choose the wholesome, homemade *manisan* over the processed, refined, commercial sweets. Their teeth are happier for it.

SHELL

1 cup pitted dates

1 cup almonds

1 cup cashews

½ cup sunflower seeds

1½ teaspoons grated lemon zest

TOPPING

3 bananas, sliced

2 cups diced papaya

1 cup diced pineapple

1 to 2 passion fruits, scooped out of shell (optional)

1 mango, peeled, pitted, and cubed (optional)

SAUCE

1 cup grated coconut

¼ cup filtered water

1 teaspoon ground cardamom

½ teaspoon fresh lemon juice

GARNISH

1 tablespoon grated coconut

2 teaspoons pine nuts

Edible flowers, such as pansies or nasturtiums

Bali Buddha Raw Tropical Pie

SERVES 4

If you're ever in Bali, just across from the post office in Ubud, you'll find a beautiful little spot called Bali Buddha that serves healthy organic food and drinks. Brenda, one of Bali Buddha's owners and the mother of three glowing daughters, shares this easy-to-make and scrumptious recipe invented by Maj Nathanson. This pie is a meal in itself: the nuts provide protein, iron, magnesium, calcium, niacin, folic acid, and vitamin E, and the tropical fruits are rich in vitamin C and thiamin (vitamin B1). If you wish to whip up something on a few minutes' notice that is so pretty it will look like you spent all day preparing it, this raw pie is the perfect treat. If you have time to soak the nuts for a few hours and rinse them, they will be very easy to digest.

To make the shell, combine the dates, nuts, seeds, and lemon zest in a food processor and blend to make a sticky paste. Press the shell ingredients into a pie plate.

To make the topping, arrange the fruit on top of the shell in any lovely fashion you like.

To make the sauce, place the coconut, water, cardamom, and lemon juice in a bowl and whisk with a fork until well-mixed. Pour the sauce over the fruit.

Garnish with the grated coconut and pine nuts, adding the flowers as a last touch. Serve immediately.

Pie Crust

MAKES 2 SINGLE OR
ONE DOUBLE 9-INCH CRUST

This recipe comes to me by way of a dear friend, Debby Nofthaft. Debby and I both lived in the small town of Fairfield, Iowa, where in the fall, the apple and pear trees are abundant with free fruit. Getting together to make pies was one of our greatest joys.

In a large bowl, mix together the flours and salt. Using a pastry cutter or fork, cut in the butter until the mixture resembles coarse crumbs.

Sprinkle the cold water over the mixture, 1 tablespoon at a time. Use a large wooden spoon to mix in the water. As you mix in the water, press the dough together, being careful not to add too much water, or the dough will become rubbery. Keep tossing the butter with the flour; this makes it flaky. This takes time; be patient. Never knead pie dough.

When the dough comes together, form it into two balls with your hands. Lightly dust a work surface with flour. Using a wooden rolling pin, roll out the dough balls, one at a time. Start from the center and roll out in all directions, adding a little extra pressure to the thicker area. Add a sprinkle of flour whenever the dough begins to stick. Pinch split edges together as needed.

When the crust is half rolled out, lift it gently and sprinkle a little more flour underneath it. Use your pie plate to determine the correct size; it will need to be a little larger than the size of the pan. Fold the rolled dough in half and gently lift it into the pie plate, then unfold.

For a single crust pie (such as for pumpkin pie), tuck the overlapping edges under so they sit on the top ledge of

I cup whole-wheat pastry flour

I cup white pastry flour

½ teaspoon sea salt

¾ cup (1½ sticks) butter, chilled

Ice water (measure out ¼ cup and drop in an ice cube)

the pie plate, flush with the edge. Shape the dough evenly and crimp the edges.

If your recipe calls for a baked pie shell (with filling to be added after baking), pierce the shell all over with many fork holes. Preheat the oven to 375°F and bake for 20 minutes, or until the shell is golden brown.

For a two-crust pie, trim the bottom crust so that it sags evenly and just a bit over the edge of the pie plate. Add the filling of your choice. Roll out the top crust and arrange over the top of filled bottom crust. Trim evenly to overlap approximately 1 inch. Tuck the top overlapped edge under the bottom crust. Pinch and crimp. Make slits in the top of the crust with a paring knife before baking.

Dessert-Making Tips

+ *N*ever cook or bake honey. Honey, a sacred food, is full of precious nutrients; it should be used raw. Add it last, to food that has cooled.

+ Look for aluminum-free baking soda and baking powder. Alcohol-free vanilla and almond extracts are available in many health-food and whole-food stores.

+ Choose organic sweeteners. Remember, a sweet tooth can be tamed when you cut out refined, commercially made sweets. After a short time of eating more healthful desserts, you will begin to enjoy desserts that are subtly sweetened.

Apple Pie

MAKES ONE 9-INCH PIE

When gathering apples in the fall, don't ignore the imperfect ones. They may have a bruise, but most of the fruit is delicious and usable. The best pie apples are a little tart and firm; Rome, Macintosh, and Golden Delicious are wonderful to use; however, don't ignore the fruit on your own trees. If you don't have fruit trees, plant one. Do it for your children and your children's children.

Prepare the pie crust according to the recipe directions for one double-crust pie.

Preheat the oven to 350°F.

In a large bowl, combine the apples (or pears or a combination of both), flour, sugar, and cinnamon, and mix well to coat the fruit. Pour the mixture into the prepared bottom crust. Cover with the top crust, seal, crimp (this is the children's job at our house) and slash the top.

Bake for about 45 minutes on a rack positioned at the center of the oven, until the crust is a beautiful golden brown. Place a cookie sheet under the pie to catch any run-off. Remove the pie from the oven and let it cool for 10 minutes before serving. If served hot, the fruit tends to run out of the slices. If you like your pie neat, serve it cooled.

Note: To make a sugarless apple pie, omit the sugar and add ½ cup raisins.

I double pie crust (see page 223)

9 cups peeled, cored, and sliced apples or pears

¼ cup whole wheat or unbleached white flour

⅓ to ½ cup raw sugar (see Note) or Sucanat

1½ teaspoons ground cinnamon

Pie crust (see page 223)

2½ cups cooked pumpkin or
   2 (16-ounce) cans
   pumpkin

1 cup raw sugar or Sucanat

2⅔ cups half-and-half

4 large eggs, beaten

4 teaspoons ground
   cinnamon

3 teaspoons ground ginger

2 teaspoons ground nutmeg

1 teaspoon ground cloves

½ cup pecan halves, for
   garnish (optional)

Traditional Pumpkin Pie

MAKES TWO 9-INCH PIE

I was born in November and love pumpkin pie so much that growing up, I often asked my mother to make it for my birthday! Pumpkin pie is a protein-rich dessert. If you can't find fresh pumpkin, organic canned pumpkin is available in most health-food stores. Cool on racks before serving with freshly whipped cream.

Prepare two single pie shells according to the recipe directions.

Preheat the oven to 350°F. Position a rack in the center of the oven.

In a large bowl, combine the pumpkin, sugar, half-and-half, eggs, cinnamon, ginger, nutmeg, and cloves, and mix well. Pour the mixture into the unbaked pie shells.

Bake for 45 to 50 minutes, or until a knife inserted into the center comes out clean. If you wish to decorate your pies beautifully, remove them from the oven after 30 minutes and arrange the pecan halves on the surface. Return the pies to the oven to finish baking.

Chay-chay's Carrot Cake

MAKES ONE 15-INCH RECTANGULAR CAKE

Chay-chay is my beloved "God-us Daughter." When her mother Alesia went into labor, it took me, Alesia's midwife, 4 minutes to go from a deep sleep to her side. Alesia labored only 1 hour and 6 minutes! Short as it was, the details of Chay-chay's birth (she came in the caul, as so many healers do) are indelibly etched on my heart. This delicious, nutritious, and egg-free dessert is her birthday cake. Our family decorates this cake with edible pansies from our garden.

Preheat the oven to 350°F.

Position a rack in the center of the oven. Grease a 15-by-10-by-2-inch rectangular baking pan and dust it lightly with flour.

In a large bowl combine the oil, sugar, and soy milk, and mix well.

In a separate bowl, sift together the flours, baking soda, baking powder, salt, cinnamon and allspice.

Add the flour mixture to the soy milk mixture and blend well. Add the carrots, nuts, and currants. Mix gently but thoroughly. Pour the mixture into the prepared baking pan.

Bake for 40 to 45 minutes, or until a cake tester inserted into the center comes out clean.

While the cake is baking, mix the topping ingredients together and beat until fluffy. Set aside. Once the cake is finished, remove from the oven to cool thoroughly before frosting with the topping.

1 cup vegetable oil

1 cup raw sugar or Sucanat

1½ cups vanilla soy milk or 1½ cups crushed pineapple in juice

2 cups unbleached all-purpose flour

2 cups whole-wheat or spelt flour (available in health-food stores)

2 teaspoons natural baking soda

2 teaspoons natural baking powder

2 teaspoons sea salt

2 teaspoons ground cinnamon

½ teaspoon ground allspice

3 cups grated carrots

1 cup chopped nuts (walnuts, pecans, blanched almonds)

½ cup currants or raisins

TOPPING

1 pound cream cheese, at room temperature

¼ cup raw honey

2 teaspoons vanilla extract or 1 tablespoon fresh lemon juice

6 large apples, such as
  Golden Delicious or
  Granny Smith, peeled and
  cored

7 teaspoons raw sugar or
  Sucanat

2 egg whites, beaten

4 teaspoons freshly
  squeezed orange juice

Baked Apples à la Sophia

SERVES 6

Leave it to a Dutch artist to come up with a simple and sublime way to indulge in apples. This is so surprisingly delicious—a sweet dream, really.

Preheat the oven to 400°F. Place the prepared apples in a buttered 9-by-13-by-2-inch baking dish. Pour 1 teaspoon of sugar into each apple's center. Bake the apples for 20 minutes.

Meanwhile beat the egg whites until fluffy with 1 teaspoon sugar and 1 teaspoon orange juice.

Decrease the oven temperature to 200°F. Remove the baked apples and pour ½ teaspoon orange juice over each apple. Top each with a dollop of beaten egg white. Return the apples to the oven, with the door slightly ajar.

Serve dinner. By the time you are ready for dessert, the apples will be perfect—not be too hot, but well done. The egg white topping will be slightly crunchy. Delightful.

Surreal's Delight

SERVES 8 TO 10

This is our family version of baklava—I always make it with maple syrup or jam rather than honey because I prefer not to cook honey. We call it Surreal's Delight because it was invented while our dear Surreal was living beside us, just when her baby brother, Into, was born. It's a not-too-sweet celebration treat. The nuts contribute the protein, vitamins, and minerals. This dessert is delicious served warm with a side of plain or vanilla yogurt.

Preheat the oven to 350°F.

To assemble the layers, using a pastry brush, lightly coat the bottom of a 9-by-13-by-2-inch baking pan with butter. Working quickly so the filo dough doesn't dry out, unroll the filo dough and loosely cover with a damp (not wet) cloth or paper towel to keep it from drying out as you work. Lay a sheet of filo in the pan, as neatly and flat as possible. Fold the filo sheet in half widthwise to make it fit in the pan. Brush with butter. Repeat this step with three sheets of filo, brushing very lightly with butter between each sheet. After you've buttered the fourth sheet of filo, drizzle about 3 tablespoons of maple syrup over it. Sprinkle ½ cup of chopped nuts over this. Add two layers of folded filo and butter, then spread the jam in an even layer over it. Add three layers of folded filo and butter. Now make another layer of maple syrup and nuts. Add three layers of folded filo and butter. Make a third layer of nuts and syrup. Add three layers of folded filo and butter. Before baking, store the top layer of filo into serving-size portions.

Bake for 50 to 60 minutes, until the top is golden brown.

½ (16-ounce) package filo dough, thawed if frozen

6 tablespoons (¾ stick) butter, melted

½ cup blueberry, raspberry, or mixed-berry jam

9 tablespoons maple syrup

1½ cups pecans or walnuts, finely chopped

¼ cup pitted prunes, chopped

¾ cup boiling filtered water

¼ cup (½ stick) butter, at room temperature

⅓ cup blackstrap molasses

⅔ cup raw sugar or Sucanat

I large egg

I (1½-inch) piece fresh ginger, peeled and grated

1½ cups whole-wheat pastry flour

I teaspoon natural baking powder

½ teaspoon natural baking soda

½ teaspoon sea salt

I teaspoon ground cinnamon

¾ teaspoon freshly grated nutmeg

¼ teaspoon ground cloves

Maui Ginger Bread

SERVES 6

The blackstrap molasses in this dessert is rich in iron, calcium, and potassium. I call it Maui Ginger Bread because I first heard of a version of this while on the island of Maui, where ginger root grows. This inspired me to use fresh ginger root rather than dried.

Preheat the oven to 350°F. Grease a 7-by-11-inch baking dish.

Combine the prunes and ¼ cup boiling water in a blender or food processor and process until smooth. Place the butter in a medium bowl and add the prune mixture. Blend until creamy. Add the molasses, sugar, egg, and ginger, and blend well.

In a separate bowl combine the flour, baking powder, baking soda, salt, cinnamon, nutmeg, and cloves.

Using a wooden spoon or spatula, fold the wet ingredients into the dry ingredients. Slowly add the remaining ½ cup boiling water, and blend until smooth. Scrape the batter into the prepared buttered baking dish.

Position the rack in the center of oven and bake for about 30 minutes, or until a cake tester inserted into the center comes out clean. Serve warm.

Judy's Chocolate Chip Banana Bread

MAKES ONE 5X9-INCH LOAF

If you ever get a chance to spend time in North Carolina, stop in at the Purple Orchid Bed and Breakfast, just outside Ashville, in the town of Burnsville. My family had a wonderful time there, and though the entire place was lovely, Judy's and David's kitchen was our favorite spot to hang out. One frosty morning Judy surprised us with this bread, hot from her oven. Besides being fun and delicious to eat, the eggs add protein and all the wholesome ingredients make it a perfect breakfast or dessert. Serve with a steaming cup of tea. We love to slather the slices with butter and enjoy them warm from the oven.

Preheat the oven to 350°F. Grease the bottom and sides of a 5-by-9-inch loaf pan and dust with flour.

In a small bowl, combine the maple syrup, eggs, and granola.

In a large bowl, sift together the flours, salt, baking powder, nutmeg, and cinnamon.

In a medium bowl, cream together the sugar and butter, then add the bananas, mashing as you go. Add the maple syrup mixture and creamed butter mixture to the dry ingredients and stir to combine. Fold in the chocolate chips and pecans. Pour the batter into the prepared loaf pan.

Bake for 50 to 60 minutes. You'll know it's done when it smells lovely and a cake tester inserted in the center comes out clean. Remove loaf from the oven and allow to cool for 3 to 5 minutes. Serve warm or cool.

1/4 cup pure maple syrup

2 large eggs, beaten

1/2 cup granola

3/4 cup spelt flour (available in health-food stores)

I cup whole-wheat flour

1/2 teaspoon sea salt

I teaspoon natural baking powder

1/2 teaspoon freshly grated nutmeg

1/4 teaspoon ground cinnamon

1/4 cup raw sugar or Sucanat

1/2 cup (I stick) butter, softened

3 large ripe or overripe bananas, mashed

1/2 cup chocolate chips

1/2 cup pecans, coarsely chopped

Mango Ice Cream

SERVES 2 TO 4

I cup cow's, soy, or rice milk

½ cup raw sugar or Sucanat

½ teaspoon ground cardamom

I cup cream

I ripe mango, peeled, pitted, and sliced

What could be more wonderful than homemade mango ice cream?

In a small saucepan warm the milk, sugar, and cardamom until the sugar has dissolved. Allow to cool. In the blender, mix the cream and sugared milk together. Add the mango last, and do not overblend; you want some of the mango to be in chunks.

Pour the mixture into ice cube trays (usually fills three trays) and freeze. Serve in cubes or put the cubes in the food processor to make smooth mango ice cream.

Basil Ice Milk

SERVES 3 TO 4

It is so much fun watching our friends become grandparents. I remember when Christopher was a young father. Now he and Leslie are grandparents. Christopher brought this recipe back from his honeymoon in France. I admit, it sounds weird, but it tastes divine. Basil is a sacred plant in India. It nourishes the respiratory, reproductive, nervous, and digestive systems. It is said to promote love and devotion in the heart; compassion, clarity, and improved memory in the mind. It's no wonder it is served as a honeymoon treat in France.

Milk (see Note)

1 to 2 generous handfuls of fresh basil leaves

¼ to ½ cup raw sugar or Sucanat

Freeze enough milk to fill two ice cube trays. Combine the frozen milk cubes, basil, and sugar in a food processor or blender and process until smooth. Serve immediately in bowls.

Note: Cow milk makes it creamy but you can use goat's milk, rice milk, or soy milk.

I cup assorted nuts
(almonds, cashews,
pecans, walnuts,
macadamias)

¼ cup sesame seeds (or
flaxseeds, or a mixture
of both)

½ cup raisins

½ cup pitted dates

Toni's Date Balls

MAKES ABOUT 2 DOZEN BALLS

These little balls of bliss are an iron-rich treat. Toni says that you must brush your teeth right after eating them, as they are sticky.

Combine ½ cup of the nuts and 2 tablespoons of the sesame seeds in a food processor and process until you have a fine mixture. Transfer the mixture to a bowl and set aside.

Combine the remaining ½ cup nuts, 2 tablespoons seeds, raisins, and dates in the food processor, and process until well-combined. This mixture will be sticky. Form the sticky mixture into marble-sized balls, and roll in the finely chopped nut and seed mixture. Pop into happy mouths.

From the Midwife Next Door

It would be wonderful if every pregnant and breastfeeding mother had a caring midwife right next door. There was a time, long ago, when nearly every village had a wise woman, a good witch. Indeed, fortunate villages had many wise witches. The families knew they could call one or more of these women in the middle of the night, when labor awakened them. Almost more importantly, before a woman's labor ever began, she could drop by, find her midwife in the garden, or in the kitchen, and ask questions. The midwife would bring a handful of nettles and red raspberry leaves out and steep a tea. The pregnant or breastfeeding woman would bring her concerns, her questions. Sometimes the two would plant some beans as they spoke. Other times a group of women would gather at the midwife's house for food and sharing.

Today, all too many women don't have a midwife. So much of the practical wisdom that passes from woman to woman, from one generation to the next, is out of their reach. Fortunately, an increasing number of women are being called to become midwives. Perhaps by the time our granddaughters are expecting babies, they will have a good witch within reach, a midwife next door.

Mothers-to-be can seek out a midwife. There are a good handful of them scattered all over the planet. They keep women's wisdom alive by sharing it, so don't be too shy to ask questions.

Naturally, if you have persistent pregnancy complaints, which do not resolve when you try the following home remedies, you should always consult your own midwife, doctor or health-care provider.

In the meantime, here are a few practical answers to the questions I am most often asked.

DURING PREGNANCY

HOW CAN I AVOID LEG CRAMPS?

Believe me, I'll never forget the painful leg cramps I suffered from during my first pregnancy. Often they would occur in the middle of the night, which was frightening, as well as excruciating. To prevent leg cramps, make sure you are getting enough sodium, calcium, magnesium, and potassium.

+ Eat bananas, citrus fruits, yogurt, cottage cheese, dark green vegetables, sea vegetables, salmon, sardines, soybeans, almonds, and sesame seeds.

+ Avoid carbonated drinks; the phosphoric acid that is routinely added to the carbonated water in most commercial sodas and soda water can interfere with your body's natural mineral balance. Naturally carbonated water is safer.

+ Place a pillow under your legs while sleeping or sitting.

+ Never point your toes while having a leg cramp. Flex your feet, as if pulling your toes upward toward your knees, for relief.

+ A hot water bottle or heating pad, applied directly to the cramping leg, can help.

+ Having a loved one firmly hold the cramping muscles, applying manual pressure (as if pressing both ends of the muscle toward each other) until the cramp subsides, also helps.

+ Walking everyday and swimming as much as you can will increase the circulation in your legs, which helps prevent cramps.

WHAT CAN I DO TO AVOID A STRANGE, RESTLESS, ACHY FEELING IN MY LEGS OR FEET?

This is sometimes due to anemia. If you suspect you need to improve your iron intake and absorption you may:

+ Drink nettle leaf tea (available in bulk and tea bags).

+ Take yellow dock tincture (available in health-food stores).

+ Drink red raspberry leaf tea (may be mixed with nettles).

✦ Increase your intake of leafy green vegetables.

✦ Eat prunes. It's best if you soak them for a while in warm water.

✦ Drink grape juice. It's best to dilute fruit juice with 50 percent water.

✦ Take organic prenatal vitamin and mineral supplements.

✦ Take an organic liquid iron supplement.

WHAT CAN I DO TO LOWER AN ELEVATED LEVEL OF GLUCOSE IN MY URINE?

If your routine prenatal urine test shows an elevated level of glucose, and you are otherwise healthy, your midwife, doctor, or health-care provider will want to rule out diabetes. The kidneys of a pregnant woman have a lower renal threshold for glucose than non-pregnant women. Many pregnant women (up to 50 percent) spill some glucose in their urine, but their blood glucose levels remain normal. In the meantime, you can take a close look at your intake of sugar. This means refined as well as natural sugars.

Many times I have found pregnant women spill sugar in their urine because they are drinking large quantities of full-strength fruit juices. I recommend diluting fruit juice at least 50 percent with water. This is wise for all people, not just pregnant women. In fact, I would never give a child full-strength fruit juice; imagine eating 9 apples in a row. Now ask yourself: Why would you want your body to take the juice of nine apples all at once? Apples, indeed apple juice, are healthy for us. However, the sugar content of a heap of apples is just too stressful for the kidneys.

More often than not, after eliminating all sugar and sweet intake for a few days, glucose will not show up in your next urine test. Also, drinking a cup of nettle tea daily will help fortify your kidneys' filtration ability.

WHAT CAN I DO TO LOWER MY BLOOD PRESSURE?

If your blood pressure is just a bit high, try eating cucumbers. It has been found that eating even one cucumber a day can help alleviate high blood pressure. I have also found that eating watermelon and drinking the water of a young coconut can reduce high blood pressure.

WHAT CAN I DO TO RELIEVE ITCHING?

Itching skin during pregnancy can be caused by hormonal changes. Also remember that in later pregnancy, your skin must stretch, which can cause itching. Dry skin can become very irritated, especially during the winter months when forced-air heating aggravates skin discomforts. To prevent skin irritation, pregnant women (and all people) should avoid mineral oil-based skin care products, as well as harsh soap and laundry products. Some women benefit from avoiding soap altogether. Read the labels; most skin products are made with mineral oil. Also rule out irritation from any recent changes in the soap or laundry products you use. Choosing the most natural kind of shampoo, soap, and laundry products is always wise, to protect your health and the environment. Since you're making a baby, begin treating your own skin like a baby's. Many women have found that applying hexane-free castor oil softens and soothes dry and scaly skin.

Itching can often be alleviated by adding unrefined virgin olive oil to your diet. Also increase your intake of foods that are rich in vitamins A and D and linolenic acids. Foods rich in vitamin A include fish liver oil, liver, vegetables, eggs, and dairy products. Sources of vitamin D are salt water fish, sunlight (no tanning, use sunscreen), vitamin D-fortified dairy products, and fish liver oil. Linolenic acid sources are flaxseed oil, evening primrose oil, and sardines.

Between 0.02 percent and 2.4 percent of pregnant women are diagnosed with a condition called pruritus gravidarum (also called PUPS), a kind of itching unique to pregnancy. It is related to elevated estrogen and progesterone levels interfering with the liver's efficiency in excreting bile salts. Onset is usually in the third trimester, and the itching is severe. Although this condition is not characterized by lesions, abrasions caused by scratching and contact with clothing can be very painful. If this happens to you, you will wish to support your liver with the following herbs:

+ Dandelion: A detoxifying herb that supports liver function.

+ Yellow dock: Relieves heat in the circulatory system; builds iron supply.

✦ Burdock: Dispels toxins via diuresis (peeing toxins out).

✦ Beets: Nourishing and supportive; promotes elimination, and cleanses the liver.

Make sure you are drinking sufficient amounts of water. See your health-care provider (midwife or doctor) and ask about using these herbs during pregnancy.

The worse case of pruritus gravidarum I have seen was treated without antihistamine drugs. The woman's back-up physician told her that he could prescribe an antihistamine, but preferred that she consult the midwife and look for a natural alternative. This young mother remarked, "I've eaten worse in this pregnancy than in my first two. I'm not surprised I developed this skin condition." She was also suffering from anemia and exhaustion because the itching was interfering with her sleep. Within hours of starting herbal therapy to support her liver and increase her iron, she had great relief and slept through the night.

WHAT CAN I DO ABOUT PAIN FROM THE BABY KICKING?

Pain from the baby kicking may be due to hypersensitivity caused by calcium and mineral deficiency. A need for more minerals also may be evident if you experience pain in the ligaments in your groin.

These foods may help you to be more comfortable:

✦ Calcium sources: organic milk, cheese, leafy greens, legumes, almonds, tofu, tempeh, sesame seed products, fish, cherries, grapefruit, guava, honeydew melon, peaches, plums, and raspberries.

✦ Magnesium sources: wheat germ, bran, whole grains, nuts, leafy greens, avocados, blackberries, cantaloupe, guava, lemons, peaches, and raspberries.

✦ Potassium sources: apricots, avocados, bananas, cantaloupe, honeydew melon, cherries, kiwi fruit, grapes, grapefruit, pineapple, and plums.

WHAT CAN I DO ABOUT CRAVINGS FOR NONFOODS?

Pica is a condition in which a person (often a child or pregnant woman) will crave and even chew and eat nonfoods, such as dirt, sand, paint chips, bits of clothing, ice, cleanser, or other usually gritty things. This condition is due to mineral deficiency. I have seen it go away quite remarkably once the person gets sufficient mineral supplements. If someone really does not find satisfaction unless she has chewed something gritty in texture, I recommend chewing prenatal vitamins. Also chewing ice often alleviates the craving, though it is not particularly good for one's teeth. Women in Asia suffering from pica feel better when they chew raw rice.

HOW CAN I RELIEVE AND AVOID INDIGESTION?

Indigestion and heartburn are two very common pregnancy complaints. Late in pregnancy your organs are crowded and when you eat, there is precious little space for this to be a comfortable experience. Many women have found that eating a little umeboshi plum paste or sipping tea with umeboshi in it really helps as it balances digestion and eliminates bloating.

If you have heartburn-like pain that is severe and unrelenting, please see your health-care provider, to rule out ulcers.

If you suffer from indigestion, avoid onions, garlic, chocolate, and cabbages. Eat many smaller meals per day, rather than three big meals. Drink plenty of water, but do this between meals, so you are not diluting your digestive juices during meals. Remember: Stress exacerbates heartburn and indigestion; a soothing home or work environment greatly helps to relieve these discomforts.

The kitchen *is* the heart of the home. Midwives are sometimes sneaky. On home visits they will find a way to peek inside your refrigerator and cupboards, to see what foods you actually keep on hand. She won't notice the mess in your house, but she'll take to heart the foods she sees. Is the food in your larder fresh and full of life? Better yet . . . is there a garden patch providing the family with life-giving vegetables, fruits, and uplifting flowers? Your midwife will advise you to stock up on wholesome foods. She will notice if your kitchen is a busy, happy place where children and neighbors gather for nourishment. We are nourished by laughter, love, sunshine, clean water, companionship, music, color, trees, and plants, as well as food.

BREASTFEEDING WISDOM

Often a new mother will call me or drop by to say, "My baby is restless. She won't sleep no matter what I do." I make her a cup of soothing chamomile tea and tell her that this is a temporary situation. Babies grow and change day by day. Eventually, both you and baby will adjust to sleeping habits that suit you both.

If you are drinking soft drinks, tea, or coffee containing caffeine (or eating chocolate, which has caffeine in it), your baby will be fussy. A baby's liver takes much longer than an adult's liver to assimilate caffeine. This means that long after you no longer feel the effects of the caffeine you drank, your baby still will be integrating the caffeine he or she got through your breast milk. Try to stay away from caffeine, but don't wean your baby to protect him from the caffeine you may be taking. Your breast milk, even if you are drinking caffeinated beverages, is a far superior food for your growing baby.

Take a nap when your baby naps. This will help you cope with the night waking. Also, make sure you are eating enough calcium- and mineral-rich foods and getting enough protein. Stress adds to your daily need for calories and nutrients. Do not forget that breastfeeding requires more calories and nutrients than pregnancy.

If your nursing baby gets a runny nose or has a lot of mucus, but seems otherwise healthy, s/he may be reacting to your diet. The most effective way I have found to reduce excessive mucus in a breastfeeding baby is to reduce the mother's intake of dairy and sugar. In fact, the combination of dairy and sugar, as in ice cream, seems especially irritating. All of my sons, as nursing babies, were sensitive to dairy and sugar, and especially to both in combination. I also found their reaction was worse if I ate a non-organic dairy product. Excessive mucus may make a baby's breathing uncomfortable. It can interrupt sleep, which is the last thing a breastfeeding mom needs. If your baby is having this kind of discomfort, eliminate dairy and sugar from your diet. Try it and see if it makes a difference.

While breastfeeding, many questions come up. I have been amazed at how very helpful it is for mothers to attend La Leche League meetings. These gatherings usually occur monthly. There are La Leche League International chapters all over the U.S. and in many parts of the world. Check their web site for a contact in your area: http://www.lalecheleague.org or email them at: lllhq@llli.org.

While pregnant and breastfeeding, and for the rest of your life, take deep breaths. Look out the window; let the view nourish you. Listen to soothing, healing music. Walk barefoot in the garden. Go swimming, dance a little, have some fun. Living a life full of gratitude helps us truly enjoy. By eating well and attaining nourishment both physically and spiritually, you will feel more balanced. Balance is the dancing foundation upon which fulfillment and contentment are built.

Appendix

THREE-DAY FOOD DIARY*

Eating wisely is the best prevention for most common complaints and major complications of pregnancy. Make copies of this three-day food diary. In your first trimester, choose any three days in a row, for each month, and write down every single thing you eat. In your second and third trimesters, fill out the three-day food diary every two weeks. This visual record will help you really get a handle on what you are eating and how often. Share it with your midwife or doctor when you go for prenatal visits. It is a wonderful tool for fine-tuning your health. Breastfeeding moms would be wise to continue keeping the three-day food diary, once a month. Keep in mind that breastfeeding requires even more additional calories than pregnancy!

Note: "Extra" means something that may not be a nutritious choice—perhaps something just for fun or comfort.

	DAY 1	DAY 2	DAY 3
BREAKFAST			
WHOLE GRAIN:			
PROTEIN:			
FRUIT/VEGETABLE:			
(EXTRA)			
MORNING SNACK			
WHOLE GRAIN:			
PROTEIN:			
FRUIT/VEGETABLE:			
LUNCH			
WHOLE GRAIN:			
PROTEIN:			
FRUIT/VEGETABLE:			
(EXTRA)			
MIDDAY SNACK			
WHOLE GRAIN:			
PROTEIN:			
FRUIT/VEGETABLE:			
DINNER			
WHOLE GRAIN:			
PROTEIN:			
FRUIT/VEGETABLE:			
(EXTRA)			
BEDTIME SNACK			
WHOLE GRAIN:			
PROTEIN:			
FRUIT/VEGETABLE:			
MIDDLE OF THE NIGHT SNACK			

(Remember, if you wake up at night and feel restless, your body may be low on nutrients. Eating protein is a great way to put your body back at ease. You'll find you fall back to sleep much more easily after a midnight or 3 a.m. snack!)

Drinks: Make sure you are imbibing enough.

At the end of each day, look over your food diary. Ask yourself the following:

+ Are you eating wholesome, quality food at *every* meal?
+ Are you eating at least two to three servings of protein, every day?
+ Is your protein from a variety of sources? (Eggs, nuts, chicken, beans, yogurt, etc.)
+ Are you using a variety of whole grains? (*Not* white rice, or white pasta; these are "extras.")
+ Are you eating leafy green vegetables every day to prevent anemia?
+ Are you eating orange-colored fruit or vegetables daily (vitamin A, the infection fighter)?
+ Are you eating at least one or two fruits or vegetables high in vitamin C every day?
+ Are you eating to satisfaction at every meal or snack? (Remember, your baby requires nutrients 24 hours a day; it is your job to provide the fuel. Your appetite will tell you when you're "low" on fuel. Please listen to it.)
+ Are you salting your food to taste? (Your body needs salt; you are making additional blood to support the pregnancy. Find your own balance, by tuning into your taste buds.)
+ Are you drinking enough water? Water is essential to life. Please drink. For optimal digestion, drink heartily between meals.

It is beneficial to include the following in your daily diet:

Essential fatty acids: flaxseed oil, nuts, nut butters, fish. This kind of fat is essential for your growing baby's brain development.

Sea vegetables: dulse, nori, kombu, kelp, etc. These provide minerals for the development and maintenance of strong bones and blood.

Nutritional yeast or another source of B-complex: In the first trimester, B vitamins help prevent birth defects. They also decrease nausea, alleviate anemia, and replace energy, which gets used up by stress.

Chlorophyll: Available in powdered form at health food stores and present in leafy green vegetables. Helps build blood and prevent anemia.

Red raspberry leaf tea: Found at health-food stores in bulk and in tea bags. A traditional uterine tonic herb. After the sixteenth week of pregnancy, it can be safely taken in generous amounts.

Pure water: Absolutely essential to all life. You must drink a minimum of 8 tall glasses of pure water, every day.

* A special thanks to Christina Wadsworth and Beverly Francis, who first made the three-day food diary for the expectant women of Iowa.

Afterword

Growing up Filipino-American meant that every meal was an international experience. There was Filipino food, which my mother, my brother Bobby, and I just loved, and then there was American-style cuisine, for my father, sister Christine and brothers Carl and Gregory. Since my mother is also half-Chinese, we often tasted China, or a "Pinoy" version of Chinese food. This was a multinational juggling act that only an excellent, energetic cook like my mother could pull off. She did this every single day, and she did it deliciously. Cresencia Lim Jehle was truly my foundation.

Of course, there was my *lola* (grandmother in Filipino, and who we called Nanang, which means mother) with whom we were fortunate enough to live much of our lives. It was Nanang who took me into the garden to pick leafy greens and dig *kamote* (sweet potato). We would hike into the forests of Baguio to gather herbs for medicine and for food. She taught me how to chase a chicken in the yard and how to prepare an egg on a wood stove made from a cut-up metal drum. It was Nanang who taught me how to make something scrumptious out of what appeared to be nothing. This she undoubtedly learned during WWII, as a refugee mother and hilot (midwife/healer).

As a teenager, I worked a season at the Uncle Mustache Falafel Stand in Isla Vista, California. I learned that you need to put plenty of tahini sauce on a falafel. I learned that simple things like tomato slices and a little pickle are just the artist's touch. I learned that I could multitask with the best of cooks: serving, frying, chopping, smiling, pouring drinks, toasting pita bread, chatting, and loving it all.

Then there was the phone call….Maharishi International University was holding a course in Isola, in the mountains between France and Italy, upcountry from Nice. They desperately needed a vegetarian cook. Three days later, I found myself on a free flight to Europe. I wasn't afraid, but I should have been. Imagine landing in Stuttgart, Germany, still a teenager, and spending the first night sleeping on a bench in a train station. I found my way to France, and eventually to Isola, which would be my home for the next few months.

Once there I found one hundred fifty hungry people who needed wholesome meals three times a day, plus snacks. That was 1975, and much of the produce was coming from Spain. Well, it stopped coming when the political climate suddenly changed upon the death of Spain's president. The Spanish borders closed, and produce headed for countless destinations all over Europe rotted on trucks and wagons. We made do for a few weeks on winter cabbage and the kindness of the neighboring farmers.

I'll never forget Mimi and Michael, twins from Germany, who at the tender age of fourteen, were our servers in Isola. It was their job to select, slice, and serve the thirty varieties of cheese we had on hand. If you've seen a wheel of Parmesan the size of a Volkswagon tire, or those tiny triangles of soft Laughing Cow, you know what an astonishing art form cheese is in Europe. Then there was Ronald, so very French: he was our pot washer, and he sang in an echoing baritone. Heiner and Ann prepared vegetables for hours. There were three Cockney guys who showed up hungry one night and joined our staff. They would do the heaviest work, with a smile. Sweet Randy kept us all guessing (what was his job?).

On the course I met Debby, a young mother expecting her second child (that would be our David). Debby was very sick with nausea, and her body was having difficulty maintaining this pregnancy. I became determined to cook something that Debby could hold down. Something simple and full of protein, as I believed that her baby would survive if only we could give him some blocks with which to build his body. Egg drop soup was the answer. As Debby's strength grew, the spotting subsided; she began to come down to the kitchen and give me pointers. She will never fully understand how profoundly she affected me. It was the way she would lovingly chop parsley, stop to sing a song to her four-year-old son, Marsten, and turn back to her task. Her whispered pointers about nutrition sparked my passion for the subject. It has been twenty-seven years since Debby and I met; we are still enjoying a deep and rewarding friendship. Our children are still best friends, though we've lived both as close neighbors, and, at other times, on opposite sides of the globe. I hope you can get a copy of Debby's cookbook, *Cabbages & Roses.*

Soon the course in Isola ended and we left for Vittel, France, with its beautiful water, in the lovely Lorraine.

I was married, and too young to be. I found myself expecting a baby: Déjà resulted. In this way, I began to focus my passion for food on my own richly growing belly.

As a gift, I had been given a beautiful macrobiotic cookbook, which was lost long ago. What I never did lose was some simple and profound advice about respecting food and preparing it with love and consciousness. This little book pointed out how precious a cooking pot really was, how sacred a bowl. I began to see pots and bowls as metaphors for women's bodies. A bountiful bowl brimming with salad or rising bread dough became a beautiful pregnant woman in my eyes.

Fast forward . . . I found myself the mother of four children, living in Maui, Hawaii. Gardening in Hawaii is food nirvana; I could lean out of my kitchen window and pick a ripe papaya. Every morning I would wake to the cry of "maaaa—ma," as my goats called me to milk them. Lizzybel, Twinkle, Josephine, and Iva Mae were wonderful companions, and generous with their milk. I'll always cherish those mornings with my daughters, Lakota and Zhòu, milking the "girls," and singing. Returning to the kitchen, we would share a warm cup of our goat's milk, and sometimes a tiny chocolate. All this just as the sun was rising in the Hawaiian sky.

I learned to dry bananas; and to make a mango smoothie, a tea from hibiscus blossoms, and a salad with starfruit slices. It was during this time that I wrote *After the Baby's Birth,* a book that was truly a labor of love. It was the letters from new mothers, praising the recipes in *After the Baby's Birth,* that inspired me to begin organizing a cookbook for pregnant and breastfeeding women and their families. This "organization" took a good fourteen years, and I'm still gathering knowledge and harvesting, inventing, and testing recipes.

Fate took husband Wil, the children, and me to Bali, where, after the birth of our son Hanoman, my work in midwifery began. Living in a village taught me so much about community. It was there I became an *ibu* (a mother of my family and my neighbors, and for a broadening global clan).

Behind our house we witnessed the cycles of growing rice, from emerald seedlings in flooded fields to waving golden ripening grain. The men planted the seeds, and the women harvested—just like the making of babies. To witness this, season after season, deepened my love affair with rice.

In Bali, the leading cause of adult death is hemorrhage after childbirth.[1] This tragic fact led me to look for solutions. I found that these deaths were preventable. The lifesaving key: proper nutrition. According to Mangku (father-priest) Liyar, my good friend, who was a *dukun bayi* (traditional birth attendant) in his younger years, the women began to hemorrhage after "modern industrialized" farming techniques were imported from the West. In particular, the indigenous red rice of Bali was replaced by "Green Revolution" rice, which grows more quickly but is sprayed with pesticides and fungicides, then polished. This new white rice did not give women the nutritional support they needed to survive pregnancy and childbirth. Life as it had slowly evolved in Bali, over centuries, had changed in one growing season. The people's staple food had been replaced with hybrid rice that could be grown quickly, using chemicals along the way. The results were devastating. Not only did the women die in alarming numbers, the otherwise healthy babies, more often than not, did not survive. They needed the mother's milk, and she was gone.

The experience of being a midwife in Bali, receiving babies in family homes, small clinics, and hospitals, gave me a profound respect for nutrition. In the words of Nan Koehler, author of *Artemis Speaks,* "Nutrition is everything for the pregnant woman and her baby."[2] Human beings, particularly women growing babies in their bellies, need clean air, pure water, shelter, happiness, and wholesome food. On planet Earth, nearly 600,000 women between the ages of fifteen and forty-nine die every year as a result of complications arising from pregnancy and childbirth.[3] If we as a global community wish to stop losing more than one mother per minute, we must make headway in the human rights issues of clean water and nutritious food. Writing this book is my small contribution toward getting the news out there. Sometimes my hands are busy receiving a baby into the world. Sometimes I suture wounds, or write words. More often, my hands are busy gardening with my granddaughter and preparing food for my family, just like your hands, dear mothers.

The research and writing of Dr. Michel Odent is alerting the world about the importance of each individual new baby, and to the fact that conditions of pregnancy, one's birth, and the first hour or two of life make the person who he or she essentially is.[4] Knowing this, every pregnant woman and her family must strive toward optimal conditions for the growing of the new baby.

The water you drink and the food you eat while expecting your baby make a tremendous difference. You can greatly improve your health and your childrens' health.

We live in our bodies; they are our "houses." Saint Francis called his body "Brother Donkey," and he learned to love and care for it as it carried him along in his spiritual work. Physical health allows us to grow intellectually and emotionally; it opens up to spread the wings of our consciousness. For the expectant mother, wholesome living is a yoga, a spiritual quest in itself, for she shares all the benefits of her improved health with her baby.

I know in my heart that each baby, each mother, each family is important. It is upon these individuals that we will build a peaceful world. It is only by giving the newest citizens of our Earth a gentle, healthy, wholesome start that we can hope for a bright future. This book is for you dear mothers, now and in the future. This book is for your babies, architects of peace.

Om Shanti. Thank you, I love you.
Ibu Robin Lim

---

[1] Inne Susante M.D. *Complications of Pregnancy and Childbirth* (a study for UNICEF in 1983).

[2] Nan Koehler, phone conversation with the author, winter 2001.

[3] World Health Organization/UNICEF/World Bank, "Reduction of Maternal Mortality: A Joint WHO/UNICEF/World Bank Statement," World Health Organization, Geneva. Report 10 of the Council on Scientific Affairs, (1999): 1 – 99.

[4] Michel Odent, M.D. *The Scientification of Love* (London and New York, Free Association Books, 1999).

Index